HEALING TRAUMA

PETER A. LEVINE, PH.D.

HEALING TRAUMA

*A Pioneering Program for
Restoring the Wisdom of Your Body*

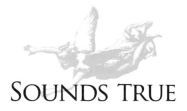

SOUNDS TRUE

Sounds True, Inc., Boulder, CO 80306
© 2005 Peter A. Levine

SOUNDS TRUE is a trademark of Sounds True, Inc.

Published 2005
Printed in Korea

ISBN 1-59179-247-9

Library of Congress Control Number: 2004117500

Audio learning programs by Peter A. Levine from Sounds True:
It Won't Hurt Forever: Guiding Your Child through Trauma
Healing Trauma: Restoring the Wisdom of the Body
Sexual Healing: Transforming the Sacred Wound

MEDICAL ALERT

You deserve to get the help you need in healing your traumas. The series of exercises presented in this book/CD is not a form of, or a substitute for, psychotherapy. If you are experiencing symptoms of trauma, you may need to enlist competent professional help. If you choose to perform these exercises on your own, and if you experience physical or emotional reactions that feel too intense to manage, you should seek professional help. You can find a list of practitioners trained in working with this approach to trauma on the web site, www.traumahealing.com.

Table of Contents

Acknowledgements

I WISH FIRST TO THANK the many people that I have worked with, for their courage and for the privilege of having let me walk with them on their journeys. In particular I am indebted to the children and babies who have graced me with their miraculous innocence and soaring spirits. Through their "child's play" they have illuminated the wisdom of the organism to heal and to become whole.

To my parents, Morris and Helen, I give thanks for the gift of life, the vehicle for the expression of my work, and for their continued full and unequivocal support from both sides of the physical plane. To Pouncer, the Dingo dog, who has been my guide into the animal world as well a constant companion, and who at the age of seventeen, joyfully, chased his last rabbit; thank you for showing me the vital joy of corporeal life.

I thank my many amazingly talented students—and colleagues—both for their support and for challenging me; particularly my appreciation goes to the dedicated teachers of Somatic Experiencing® for continuing to bring this work into the world.

I thank, especially, my dear friend Maggie Kline for her generous help and support for this and other projects. In addition, I offer appreciation to Maureen Harrington for her help. I also thank Mitchell Clute of Sounds True, for his artful production, as well as Alice Feinstein and the other production people at Sounds True for their creativity and professionalism. And, finally, my gratitude is to Tami Simon for her vision and ongoing support in bringing these ideas and tools to the public.

I thank, finally, fate, destiny, synchronicity, or even blind luck and coincidence for my unusual path in life and work. I have had the opportunity and honor to share such deep and rich experiences with so many of my clients, students, and colleagues over these many short years.

—PETER A. LEVINE, PH.D.

Introduction: A Tiger Shows the Way

FOR THE LAST 35 YEARS, I have been studying stress and trauma, as well as helping people heal from its effects. I am often asked how I can work with a subject as morbid as trauma without becoming burned out or depressed. My answer to this question is that witnessing the transformation that takes place in people when they master their traumas has proven to be a deeply sustaining and uplifting experience in my life. How can that be?

Let me begin by telling you a little about myself. I began my career as a scientist in the radical environment of Berkeley, California, in the mid-1960s. While studying the effects of accumulated stress on the nervous system, I began to suspect that most organisms have an innate capacity to rebound from threatening and stressful events. At that time, I had no knowledge of psychological trauma—the term would not be defined in its modern form for another 15 years.

I was experimenting with different stress reduction techniques that employed the "new" idea of a mind/body connection.

During this early research, a singular event occurred that would forever change the direction of my work. A psychiatrist who was familiar with my stress research asked me to see a patient of his who was suffering from various "psychosomatic" symptoms, such as migraines, PMS, chronic pain, and fatigue, as well as severe panic attacks. The psychiatrist thought that this patient would benefit from learning how to relax her body.

As I began working with this patient (let's call her "Nancy"), she began to relax. Suddenly, without warning, she panicked. Terrified, and with no notion of what to do, I saw in my mind's eye the fleeting image of a tiger poised for attack. It appeared dreamlike, and, at that time, I had no idea where it had come from.

"There's a tiger coming after you, Nancy," I blurted out without thinking. *"Run and escape to those rocks. Run for your life!"* To my amazement, Nancy's body began to shake and tremble. Her cheeks flushed red as she started to sweat profusely. After several minutes, she took a few spontaneous deep breaths. This response, which was scary for both of us, washed over her in waves for almost an hour. At the end she experienced a profound calm, saying she felt "held in warm tingly waves."

Nancy reported to me that during this hour she saw mental pictures of herself at age four being held down and given ether anesthesia for a tonsillectomy. The fear of suffocation she experienced as a child—and that she remembered and revisited during her session with me—was terrifying. As a child she had felt overwhelmed and helpless. After this one session with me, her whole host of debilitating symptoms improved dramatically, and she was able to get on with her life.

That experience with Nancy changed the course of my life. Ultimately, it opened new avenues in my ongoing research into the nature of stress and trauma, deepened my understanding of how trauma affects the body, and led to a whole new way of treating the debilitating after-effects that can take so many negative and destructive forms.

The effects of unresolved trauma can be devastating. It can affect our habits and outlook on life, leading to addictions and poor decision-making. It can take a toll on our family life and interpersonal relationships. It can trigger real physical pain, symptoms, and disease. And it can lead to a range of self-destructive behaviors. But trauma doesn't have to be a life sentence.

As a result of my years of research and clinical work, I've developed an approach using physical and mental exercises that can help cleanse the body and mind of the debilitating effects of trauma. Over the last 30 years, I have witnessed transformation in the lives of literally *thousands* of people as they healed from traumatic events.

This is the Twelve-Phase Healing Trauma Program that I will be sharing with you in the rest of this book and in the accompanying CD. Using this program, you begin the healing process on Day One. And as you continue using the program in the weeks and months to come, you should experience a gradual healing process that helps you free your body and mind from the debilitating long-term symptoms of trauma.

Before we get to the details of how the program works, however, it will be helpful for you to know a little more about what trauma is and exactly how it gets into the body and causes such a wide variety of symptoms. In the brief overview presented in the opening chapters of this book, I give you what you need to know in order to understand this program—how and why it works.

Before beginning the exercises, it's important that you read all the preceding material in the book. If you're familiar with what trauma is and how it can affect you, the exercises are much more likely to have a powerfully positive effect on your unresolved trauma.

I go into a great deal more detail about my research and the physiology of trauma in my bestselling book *Waking the Tiger: Healing Trauma* (North Atlantic Books, 1997).

If you would like to read more about theory and personal case examples, if you want to know more about the science of why this program works, I refer you to that book. That book also features a number of inspiring stories about people who have experienced significant healing from their own past traumas. I'd like to reassure you, however, that you'll find right here in this book all that you'll need to know to make the Twelve-Phase Healing Trauma Program work for you.

THERE'S ONE MORE THING I'D LIKE
TO SHARE WITH YOU BEFORE WE BEGIN

In virtually every spiritual tradition, suffering is seen as a doorway to awakening. In the West, this connection can be seen in the biblical story of Job, as well as the dark night of the soul in medieval mysticism. The transformative power of suffering finds perhaps its clearest expression in the Four Noble Truths espoused by the Buddha. Though suffering and trauma are not identical, the Buddha's insight into the nature of suffering can provide a powerful mirror for examining the effects of trauma in your life. The Buddha's basic teaching offers guidance for healing our trauma and recovering a sense of wholeness.

The first truth, Buddha taught his disciples, is that suffering is part of the human condition. If we simply try to avoid confronting painful experiences, there is no way to begin the healing process. In fact, this denial creates the very conditions that promote and prolong *unnecessary* suffering.

The second noble truth states that we must discover *why* we are suffering. We must cultivate the courage to look deeply, with clarity and courage, into our own suffering. We often hold the tacit assumption that all of our suffering stems from events in the past. But, whatever the initial seed of trauma, the deeper truth is that our suffering is more closely a result of how we deal with the *effect* these past events have on us *in the present*.

The third noble truth holds that suffering can be transformed and healed. For those of us who have been traumatized, this can be a monumental leap of faith, but we *can* recover from trauma; indeed, my experience assisting others to heal from trauma has shown me this recovery is innate.

The fourth noble truth states that, once you have identified the cause of your suffering, you must find an appropriate path. I believe that the exercises I've developed and that you'll be learning in the Twelve-Phase Healing Trauma Program can serve as the path to lead you out of suffering and help you recapture the simple wonders of life.

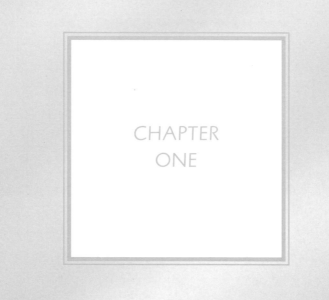

CHAPTER
ONE

What Is Trauma?

TRAUMA IS THE MOST AVOIDED, ignored, denied, misunderstood, and untreated cause of human suffering. When I use the word *trauma*, I am talking here about the often debilitating symptoms that many people suffer from in the aftermath of *perceived* life-threatening or overwhelming experiences. Recently, *trauma* has been used as a buzzword to replace everyday stress, as in, "I had a traumatic day at work." However, this use is completely misleading. While it is true that all traumatic events are stressful, all stressful events are not traumatic.

UNIQUE TO EACH INDIVIDUAL

When it comes to trauma, no two people are exactly alike. What proves harmful over the long term to one person may be exhilarating to another. There are many factors involved in the wide range of response to threat. These responses depend upon genetic make-up, an individual's history of trauma, even his or her family dynamics. It is vital that we appreciate these differences. Simply knowing that certain kinds of early childhood experiences can severely diminish our ability to cope and be present in the world may elicit compassion and support rather than harsh judgment, both for ourselves and for others.

Perhaps the most important thing I have learned about trauma is that people, especially children, can be overwhelmed by what we usually think of as common everyday events. Until recently, our understanding of trauma was limited to "shell-shocked" soldiers who have been devastated by war, victims of severe abuse or violence, and those who have suffered catastrophic accidents and injuries. This narrow view could not be further from the truth.

The fact is that, over time, a series of seemingly minor mishaps can have a damaging effect on a person. *Trauma does not have to stem from a major catastrophe.* Some common triggering events include:

- Automobile accidents (even fender benders)
- Routine invasive medical procedures
- Loss of loved ones
- Natural disasters, such as earthquakes and hurricanes

Even falling off a bicycle can be overwhelming to a child under certain circumstances. We will discuss those circumstances later. For now, I will simply say that almost all of us have experienced some form of trauma, either directly or indirectly.

For this reason, I sincerely believe that just about everyone can benefit from doing the Twelve-Phase Healing Trauma Program that you'll find in this book and on the accompanying CD.

People often ask me to define *trauma*. After thirty years, this is still a challenge. What I do know is that we become traumatized when our ability to respond to a *perceived* threat is in some way overwhelmed. This inability to adequately respond can impact us in obvious ways, as well as ways that are subtle.

Trauma can, in fact, impact us in ways that don't show up for years. For example, a traumatized war veteran who jumps every time a car backfires is clearly responding to gunfire that he experienced in the past. When a person who suffered torture and confinement breaks out in a cold sweat while riding in a crowded elevator, it is also easy to see the link. However, many, if not most of us, who have been overwhelmed by a series of less dramatic events have responses that are not so obvious.

In short, trauma is about loss of connection—to ourselves, to our bodies, to our families, to others, and to the world around us. This loss of connection is often hard to recognize, because it doesn't happen all at once. It can happen slowly, over time, and we adapt to these subtle changes sometimes without even noticing them. These are the hidden effects of trauma, the ones most of us keep to ourselves. We may simply sense that we do not feel quite right, without ever becoming fully aware of what is taking place; that is, the gradual undermining of our self-esteem, self-confidence, feelings of well-being, and connection to life.

Our choices become limited as we avoid certain feelings, people, situations, and places. The result of this gradual constriction of freedom is the loss of vitality and potential for the fulfillment of our dreams.

A NEW LOOK AT HEALING

The field of psychiatric medicine has chosen to view many of the long-term effects of trauma as an incurable disease, only marginally controllable by drugs or through behavioral management. I do not agree. While medications can at times be quite helpful, they are—of themselves—insufficient.

In working with trauma for over three decades, I have come to the conclusion that human beings are born with an innate capacity to triumph over trauma. I believe not only that trauma is curable, but that the healing process can be a catalyst for profound awakening—a portal opening to emotional and genuine spiritual transformation. I have little doubt that as individuals, families, communities, and even nations, we have the capacity to learn how to heal and prevent much of the damage done by trauma. In so doing, we will significantly increase our ability to achieve both our individual and collective dreams.

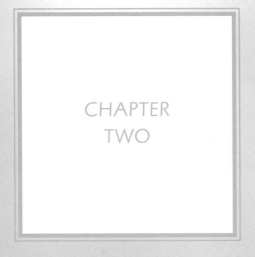

CHAPTER
TWO

The Causes and Symptoms of Trauma

BEFORE YOU BEGIN to work with the guided exercises to assist you in resolving the effects of trauma in your own life, it's useful to have an understanding of the possible causes of trauma, and to identify the various symptoms that may have arisen as a result.

Trauma is trauma, no matter what caused it. To really understand this, we need to really home in on the fact that people can be traumatized by any event they *perceive* (consciously or unconsciously) to be life-threatening. This perception is based on a person's age, life experience, and even their constitutional temperament. For example, sudden loud noises, such as thunder or the angry shouts of adults, can traumatize infants and young children. Of course, thunder and shouting are rarely life-threatening, but, when it comes to trauma, the critical factor is the *perception* of threat and the incapacity to deal with it.

CATEGORIES OF TRAUMA

The causes of trauma can be divided into two main categories—the obvious and the less obvious.

OBVIOUS CAUSES OF TRAUMA INCLUDE:

- War
- Severe childhood emotional, physical, or sexual abuse
- Neglect, betrayal, or abandonment during childhood
- Experiencing or witnessing violence
- Rape
- Catastrophic injuries and illnesses

Less obvious causes of trauma include a wide variety of seemingly ordinary events. Many of these events prove traumatizing far more often than we might expect. For that reason, I'd like you to read the following list slowly and pay special attention to your responses to each item. I want you to begin to become aware of your own "felt sense" of the things you experience. So pay special attention to your body sensations, such as tingling, muscle tightening or loosening, your breathing, and any increase or decrease in heart rate, temperature, etc.

You might also perceive fleeting images. Different colors or shapes may appear in your inner field of vision. You may have strong thoughts, memories, or emotions bubble up. On the other hand, you may experience very little, if any, response. The things I want you to pay attention to are those things that occur spontaneously. Whatever happens, I want you to try to notice it objectively, almost as if you were an outside observer. Make a mental note of it, and move on.

LESS OBVIOUS POTENTIAL CAUSES OF TRAUMA INCLUDE:

- Minor automobile accidents (even fender benders), especially those that result in whiplash

- Invasive medical and dental procedures, particularly when performed on children who are restrained or anesthetized (The use of ether increases the chance of trauma. For adults, many medical procedures, such as a pelvic exam, can be experienced as an attack, even if rationally we know they are necessary and helpful.)
- Falls and other so-called minor injuries, especially when children or elderly people are involved (for example, a child falling off a bicycle)
- Natural disasters, including earthquakes, hurricanes, tornadoes, fires, and floods
- Illness, especially where there is high fever or accidental poisoning
- Being left alone, especially in young children and babies
- Prolonged immobilization, especially in children (casting, splinting for long periods used for scoliosis or turned-in feet)
- Exposure to extreme heat or cold, especially in children and babies
- Sudden loud noises, especially in children and babies
- Birth stress, for both mother and infant

LISTEN TO YOUR BODY

How did you respond when you read the list? Did you feel a little nervous just reading the different things that can be traumatic? If so, what you are experiencing is a normal response to being reminded of things that may have been distressing to you in the past. It's not uncommon to have a couple of possible reactions. You may sense an immediate response, like a tightening in your gut, or a pounding heart. Or you may have not noticed anything while reading, but once finished, felt a slight twinge in your stomach. Or you may just have had a memory of yourself falling off of a bike without being aware of any reaction in your body.

It's very important to understand that nervousness or anxiousness, or almost any response you might have, has to do with the arousal or activation of the energy you experienced during the original overwhelming event. When you are threatened, your body instinctively generates a lot of energy to help you defend yourself against the threat. This is the energy we work with in the healing of trauma, so we need to be aware of it.

In the next chapter, I'll go into detail about how the unused energy aroused when you are threatened can get frozen into your body and cause problems and symptoms even years later.

For now, I'd like to focus on the kinds of symptoms that unresolved trauma can and often does produce.

SYMPTOMS AND THEIR ORDER OF APPEARANCE

To begin with, I want to emphasize how important it is that we view these common symptoms of trauma for what they truly are. When our bodies are feeling uneasy, they give us messages. The purpose of these messages is to inform us that something inside doesn't feel right, and it needs our attention. If these messages go unanswered, over time, they evolve into the symptoms of trauma.

It's also important to note that not all these symptoms are caused exclusively by trauma, nor has everyone who exhibits one or more of these symptoms been traumatized. The flu, for instance, can cause abdominal discomfort that is similar to trauma symptoms. However, there is a difference. Symptoms produced by the flu generally go away in a few days. Those produced by trauma do not.

The first symptoms that are likely to develop immediately after an overwhelming event include hyperarousal, constriction, dissociation and denial, as well as feelings of helplessness, immobility, or freezing. Let's take a look at each of these in turn.

Hyperarousal. This may take the form of physical symptoms—increase in heart rate, sweating, difficulty breathing (rapid, shallow, panting, etc.), cold sweats, tingling, and muscular tension. It can also manifest as a mental process in the form of increased repetitious thoughts, racing mind, and worry.

If we allow ourselves to acknowledge these thoughts and sensations, in other words let them have their natural flow, they will peak, then begin to diminish and resolve. As this process occurs, we may experience trembling, shaking, vibration, waves of warmth, fullness of breath, slowed heart rate, warmth, relaxation of the muscles, and an overall feeling of relief, comfort, and safety.

Constriction. When we respond to a life-threatening situation, hyperarousal is initially accompanied by constriction in our bodies and a narrowing of perceptions. Our nervous system acts to ensure that all our efforts can be maximally focused on the threat in an optimum way. Constriction alters a person's breathing, muscle tone, and posture in order to promote efficiency and strength. Blood vessels in the skin, extremities, and internal organs constrict so that more blood is available to the muscles, which are tensed and prepared to take defensive action. At the same time, the digestive system is inhibited. We may also feel numb and shut down.

Dissociation and denial. Woody Allen said, "I'm not afraid of dying. I just don't want to be there when it happens." This quip is a fairly accurate description of the role played by dissociation. It protects us from being overwhelmed by escalating arousal, fear, and pain. It "softens" the pain of severe injury by secreting nature's internal opium, the *endorphins.* In trauma, dissociation seems to be a favored means of enabling a person to endure experiences that are at the moment beyond endurance.

Denial is probably a lower level energy form of dissociation. The disconnection may occur between the person and the memory of or feelings about a particular event (or series of events). We may deny that an event occurred, or we may act as though it was unimportant. For instance, when someone we love dies, or when we are injured or violated, we may act as though nothing has happened, because the emotions that come with truly acknowledging the situation are too painful. In addition, dissociation may be experienced as part of the body being disconnected or almost absent. Frequently, chronic pain represents a part of the body that has been dissociated.

Feelings of helplessness, immobility, and freezing. If hyperarousal is the nervous system's accelerator, a sense of overwhelming helplessness is its brake. The helplessness that is experienced at such times is not the ordinary sense of helplessness that can affect anyone from time to time. It is the sense of being collapsed, immobilized, and utterly helpless. It is not a perception, belief, or a trick of the imagination. It is real.

SYMPTOMS: A LENGTHY LIST

Other early symptoms that begin to show up at the same time or shortly after those we just talked about can include:

- Hypervigilance (being "on guard" at all times)
- Intrusive imagery or flashbacks
- Extreme sensitivity to light and sound
- Hyperactivity
- Exaggerated emotional and startle responses
- Nightmares and night terrors
- Abrupt mood swings (rage reactions or temper tantrums, frequent anger, or crying)
- Shame and lack of self-worth
- Reduced ability to deal with stress (easily and frequently stressed out)
- Difficulty sleeping

Several of these symptoms can also show up later, even years later. Remember, this list is not for diagnostic purposes. It is a guide to help you get a feel for how trauma symptoms behave. The next symptoms that may appear are:

- Panic attacks, anxiety, and phobias
- Mental "blankness" or spaced-out feelings
- Avoidance behavior (avoiding places, activities, movements, memories, or people)
- Attraction to dangerous situations
- Addictive behaviors (overeating, drinking, smoking, etc.)
- Exaggerated or diminished sexual activity
- Amnesia and forgetfulness
- Inability to love, nurture, or bond with other individuals
- Fear of dying or having a shortened life
- Self-mutilation (severe abuse, self-inflicted cutting, etc.)
- Loss of sustaining beliefs (spiritual, religious, interpersonal)

The final group of symptoms are those that generally take longer to develop. In most cases, they may have been preceded by some of the earlier symptoms. However, there is no fixed rule that dictates when and if a symptom will appear. This group includes:

- Excessive shyness
- Diminished emotional responses
- Inability to make commitments
- Chronic fatigue or very low physical energy
- Immune system problems and certain endocrine problems such as

thyroid malfunction and environmental sensitivities
- Psychosomatic illnesses, particularly headaches, migraines, neck and back problems
- Chronic pain
- Fibromyalgia
- Asthma
- Skin disorders
- Digestive problems (spastic colon)
- Severe premenstrual syndrome
- Depression and feelings of impending doom
- Feelings of detachment, alienation, and isolation ("living dead" feelings)
- Reduced ability to formulate plans

The symptoms of trauma can be stable, that is, ever-present. They can also be unstable, meaning that they can come and go and be triggered by stress. Or they can remain hidden for decades and suddenly surface. Usually, symptoms do not occur individually, but come in groups. They often grow increasingly complex over time, becoming less and less connected with the original trauma experience.

THE COMPULSION TO REPEAT

There's one more symptom we need to look at before looking at how trauma actually gets into the body and mind and causes long-term problems. This one is a little less straightforward than the others. Here's one of the more unusual and problem-creating symptoms that can develop from unresolved trauma: the compulsion to repeat the actions that caused the problem in the first place.

We are inextricably drawn into situations that replicate the original trauma in both obvious and less obvious ways. The prostitute or stripper with a history of childhood sexual abuse is a common example. We may find ourselves re-experiencing the effects of trauma either through physical symptoms or through a full-blown interaction with the external environment.

Re-enactments may be played out in intimate relationships, work situations, repetitive accidents or mishaps, and in other seemingly random events. They may also appear in the form of bodily symptoms or psychosomatic diseases. Children who have had a traumatic experience will often repeatedly recreate it in their play. As adults, we are often compelled to re-enact our early traumas in our daily lives. The mechanism is similar regardless of the individual's age.

Bessel van der Kolk, a psychiatric researcher who has made great contributions to the field of post-traumatic stress, relates a story about a veteran that illustrates vividly both the dangerous and repetitive aspects of re-enactment in its drive toward resolution.

On July fifth in the late 1980s, a man walked into a convenience store at 6:30 in the morning. Holding his finger in his pocket to simulate a gun, he demanded that the cashier give him the contents of the cash register. Having collected about five dollars in change, the man returned to his car, where he remained until the police arrived. When the police arrived, the young man got out of his car and, with his finger again in his pocket, announced that he had a gun and that everyone should stay away from him. Luckily for him, he was taken into custody without being shot.

At the police station, the officer who looked up the man's record discovered that he had committed six other so-called "armed robberies" over the past fifteen years, all of them at 6:30 in the morning on July fifth! Upon learning that the man was a Vietnam veteran, the police surmised that this event was more than mere coincidence. They took him to a nearby VA hospital, where Dr. van der Kolk had the opportunity to speak with him.

Dr. van der Kolk asked the man directly: "What happened to you on July fifth at 6:30 in the morning?"

He responded immediately. While he was in Vietnam, the man's platoon had been ambushed by the Viet Cong. Everyone had been killed except for himself and his friend, Jim. The date was July fourth. Darkness fell and the helicopters were unable to evacuate them. They spent a terrifying night together huddled in a rice paddy surrounded by the Viet Cong. At about 3:30 in the morning, Jim was hit in the chest by a Viet Cong bullet. He died in his friend's arms at 6:30 on the morning of July fifth.

After returning to the States, every July fifth (that he did not spend in jail), the man had re-enacted the anniversary of his friend's death. In the therapy session with Dr. van der Kolk, the vet experienced grief over the loss of his friend. He then made the connection between Jim's death and the compulsion he felt to commit the robberies. Once he became aware of his feelings and the role the original event had played in driving his compulsion, the man was able to stop re-enacting this tragic incident.

What was the connection between the robberies and the Vietnam experience? By staging the robberies, the man was re-creating the fire-fight that had resulted in the death of his friend (as well as the rest of his platoon). By provoking the police to join in the re-enactment, the vet had orchestrated the cast of characters needed to play the role of the Viet Cong. He did not want to hurt anyone, so he used his fingers instead of a gun. He then brought the situation to a climax and was able to elicit the help he needed to heal his psychic wounds. That act enabled him to resolve his anguish, grief, and guilt about his buddy's violent death and the horrors of war.

If we look at this man's behaviors without knowing anything about his past, we might think he was mad. However, with a little history, we can see that his actions were a brilliant attempt to resolve a deep emotional scar. His re-enactment took him to the very edge, again and again, until he was finally able to free himself from the overwhelming nightmare of war.

ACCIDENTS "JUST" HAPPEN

Admittedly, the story of the man staging robberies every year on the same day is a rather extreme example. It serves the purpose of illustrating the fact that we can go to great lengths to create situations that will force us to confront and deal with our unresolved trauma.

Unfortunately, the link between a re-enactment and the original situation may not be readily obvious. A traumatized person may associate the traumatic event with another situation and repeat that situation instead of the original one. Recurring accidents are one common way this type of re-enactment occurs, especially when the accidents are similar in some way. In other cases, the person may continue to incur a particular type of injury. Sprained ankles, wrenched knees, whiplash, and even many so-called psychosomatic diseases are common examples of physical re-enactments.

Commonly, none of these so-called "accidents" appear to be anything but accidents. The clue to identifying them as symptoms of trauma lies in the frequency with which they occur. One young man, sexually abused as a child, had over a dozen rear-end collisions within a period of three years. In none of these "accidents" was he obviously at fault.

Frequent re-enactment is the most intriguing and complex symptom of trauma. This phenomenon can be custom-fit to the individual, with a startling level of "coincidence" between the re-enactment and the original situation. While some of the elements of re-enactment are understandable, others seem to defy rational explanation.

Let me share with you the story of Jack as an example of re-enactment that led to an accident. Jack is a very shy and serious man in his mid-fifties who lives in the Northwest. When we first met, he was quite embarrassed about his reason for seeing me. However, underneath this embarrassment was a pervasive sense of humiliation and defeat.

The previous summer, while docking his boat, he proudly and playfully announced to his wife, "Is this a beautiful job or what?" The next moment he, his wife, and their child found themselves on their backs. Jack had left the motor idling in neutral as he moored the boat, and one of the lines had gotten caught in the throttle-clutch. Suddenly, the boat lurched forward. Jack and his family were jerked off their feet.

Fortunately, no one was seriously hurt, but he smashed into another boat, causing $5,000 worth of damage. Adding insult to injury, the completely humiliated Jack got into a shouting match with the marina owner when the man (probably thinking that Jack was drunk) insisted on docking Jack's boat for him. Being an experienced boatman from a nautical family, this episode had more than knocked the wind out of him. Jack had known better than to let the engine idle while docking.

As we worked together, the underlying trauma he was re-enacting become clear. Through the felt sense—a technique we'll be using in the Twelve-Phase Healing Trauma Program—Jack was able to experience holding the rope and feeling it wrench across his burning arms before he fell on his back. This stimulated an image of himself at age five. While boating with his parents, he had fallen off a ladder onto his back. The wind was knocked out of him, and he was terrified because he could not breathe.

In exploring and remembering this early experience, Jack vividly sensed his powerful five-year-old muscles gripping onto the ladder as he proudly climbed it. His parents, being otherwise occupied, didn't see him playing on the ladder. When a large wave tipped the boat, Jack was thrown on his back. In a humiliating sequel, he was taken from doctor to doctor, repeating the story to each.

There is an important relationship between these two events—the fall at age five and his recent fiasco. In both instances he was proudly displaying his prowess in play. In both events he was thrown on his back, having the wind literally and emotionally knocked out of him. His father's boat was called *The High Seas*. A week prior to the mishap, Jack had christened his own boat *The High Seas*.

With this story in mind, you might look for events and/or accidents in your own life that seem strangely repetitious, as they may well show the mark of some unresolved trauma. Perhaps you have entirely forgotten the original event that initiated the pattern of behavior you revisit through re-enactment. Often, when exploring these possible re-enactments, you'll get a sense of both knowing and not knowing. As you work with these patterns and the memories they may awaken, trust your own felt sense and give yourself the freedom to explore the hidden connections.

Curiously, yet another symptom that can develop is avoidance. If you fell off a ladder as a child, you might forever be compelled to avoid ladders and not even begin to understand where your aversion is coming from.

SYMPTOMS DELIVER A MESSAGE

It is important to understand that any or all of these symptoms can appear no matter what kind of event caused the trauma. And these symptoms can and will disappear when the trauma is healed. In order to heal trauma, we need to learn to trust the messages our bodies are giving us. The symptoms of trauma are internal wake-up calls. If we learn how to listen to these calls, how to increase the awareness of our bodies, and, finally, how to use these messages, we can begin to heal our traumas. So if you are upset in reading these symptoms, you can perhaps re-frame your reaction as the initial phases in your healing journey. You might, instead, be grateful that your body is sending you messages that healing needs to happen.

CHAPTER THREE

Oh, Lord, help me to be a good animal today.

—Barbara Kingsolver

How Trauma Affects the Body

EARLY ON IN MY STUDY OF TRAUMA, I was involved in brain research. I knew that the instinctive parts of both human and animal brains are virtually identical. Only the rational part of our brain is uniquely human. I also knew that prey animals in the wild, though routinely threatened, are rarely traumatized. Rather, they seem to have a built-in ability to literally shake off the effects of life-threatening encounters, and go on with their lives almost as if nothing unusual had happened.

While studying footage of wild prey animals, I noticed that most animals have a similar physiological process for returning to normal after a narrow escape from death. This process was uncannily reminiscent of the shaking, trembling, and spontaneous breathing that I had watched Nancy move through. (You'll recall that you met Nancy in the introduction to this book.) I had also observed this process in many shamanic healing rituals performed throughout the world.

You can watch an example of this process from beginning to end on the *National Geographic* video "Polar Bear Alert," available at many video stores. In this video, a frightened bear is chased down by an airplane, shot with a tranquilizer dart, surrounded by wildlife biologists, and then tagged.

As the massive animal comes out of its state of shock, it begins to tremble lightly. The trembling intensifies steadily, then peaks into a near-convulsive shaking—its limbs flail seemingly at random. After the shaking stops, the animal takes deep, organic breaths that spread throughout its body. The biologist narrator of the film comments that the behavior of the bear is necessary because it "blows off stress" accumulated during the chase and capture.

Now here's the interesting part: When the bear's response is viewed in slow motion, it becomes obvious that the seemingly random leg gyrations are actually coordinated running movements. It is as though the animal *completes its escape* by actively finishing the running movements that were interrupted at the moment when it was tranquilized. Then, the bear shakes off the "frozen energy" as it surrenders in spontaneous, full-bodied breaths—just as I had observed with Nancy in her recovery from being overwhelmed as a young child.

As the evidence mounted, I grew increasingly convinced that the healing of trauma—whether it is called "re-association" or, as shamans refer to it, "soul retrieval"—is primarily a biological process or bodily process often accompanied by psychological effects. This is especially true when the trauma involved betrayal by those who were supposed to protect us. Additionally, I surmised that successful healing methods inevitably involve establishing a connection to the body. Those methods that do not enable people to reconnect with their bodies invariably have limited success.

Now let's put it all together.

FIGHT, FLIGHT, AND FREEZE

When a situation is perceived to be life-threatening, both mind and body mobilize a vast amount of energy in preparation to fight or escape—that's why this is known as the "fight or flight" response. This is the same energy that can enable a slight-framed woman to lift a ton of Detroit steel off of her son's legs when her little one is trapped under a car. This kind of strength is supported by a large increase in blood to the muscles, and the release of stress hormones, such as cortisol and adrenaline.

In the act of lifting 2,000 pounds, the mother discharges most of the excess chemicals and energy she mobilized to deal with the threat. Her son, who was trapped beneath the car, immobilized by pain and fear, would be unable to do so. This discharge of energy from the body, when complete, informs the brain that it is time to reduce the levels of stress hormones—that the threat is no longer present. This is what happens to the mother in a case like this.

If this message to normalize is not given, the brain just continues to release high levels of adrenaline and cortisol, and the body holds onto its high-energy, ramped-up state. This is the situation the son faces. Unless he can find a way to discharge the excess energy, his body will keep responding as if it were in pain and helpless, long after he has recovered from his physical injuries. The central question is: What prevents people from returning to normal functioning after a threat no longer exists? Why can't we simply release our excess energy the way animals naturally do?

To answer this question, I invite you to visit the Serengeti Plain that dwells in the ancient shadows of our psyches. Take a moment to visualize a crouching chee-tah, its eyes focused, its muscles twitching in anticipation, as it prepares to attack a swift, darting impala. I want you to track your own responses as you watch the sleek cheetah overtake its prey in a seventy-mile-an-hour surge of speed. The impala falls to the ground an instant before the cheetah sinks its claws into the haunches of its prey. It is almost as if the animal has surrendered itself to the predator and to certain death.

However, the fallen impala is not dead. Although it appears limp and motion-less, its nervous system is still highly charged from the swift chase. Though it is barely breathing or moving, the animal's heart and brain are still racing. The same chemicals discussed earlier that helped fuel its attempted escape continue to flood its brain and body. There is a possibility that the impala will not be devoured immediately. The mother cheetah may drag its (apparently dead) prey behind a bush, then go seek out its hungry cubs, safely hidden at a distance.

While the cheetah is gone, the temporarily "frozen" impala may awaken from its state of shock, then shake and tremble in order to discharge the vast amount of energy it mobilized to escape death. After completing this normalization procedure, the impala will stand up on wobbly legs, take a few tentative steps, then bound off in search of the herd as if nothing unusual had occurred.

The "immobility response" used by the impala is just as important a survival tool as "fight" and "flight." This normal survival strategy is also called the "freezing" response. Slow and relatively unprotected animals like the opossum use immobility as their first line of defense. Any animal that is trapped in a situation where fight and flight are not viable options will use it.

Another of the vital functions of the immobility response is numbness. If the impala (or human) is killed while "frozen," it will not suffer pain or even terror during its demise.

We humans use the immobility response—frozen energy—regularly when we are injured or even when we feel overwhelmed. Unlike the impala, though, we tend to have trouble returning to normal after being in this state. The very feelings that we need to access in order to us help steer ourselves back to the present are, in effect, numbed-out.

This difficulty in normalizing ourselves is very important. I believe that the ability to return to equilibrium and balance, after using the "immobility response," is the primary factor in avoiding being traumatized.

How do wild animals successfully return to their normal state?

The answer likes in the particular type of spontaneous shaking, trembling, and breathing that I described earlier. I remember that when I shared my observations about animal behavior with Andrew Bwanali, chief park biologist of the Mzuzu Environmental Center in Malawi, Central Africa, he nodded excitedly, then burst out: "Yes ... yes ... yes! That is true. Before we release captured animals back into the wild, we make absolutely sure that they have done just what you have described."

He looked down at the ground, then added softly, "If they have not trembled and breathed that way before they are released, they will not survive. They will die."

Although humans rarely die from trauma, if we do not resolve it, our lives can be severely diminished by its effects. Some people have even described this situation as a "living death."

So, why can't we shake off the immobility response, just as the animals do? What's to stop us from releasing that frozen energy?

There's some really good news here. My research led me to believe that there is every reason to believe that people do, in fact, possess the same built-in ability to shake off threat that animals do. And in my clinical practice, I have found this to be the case. I found that, if given appropriate guidance, human beings can and do shake off the effects of overwhelming events and return to their lives using exactly the same procedures that animals use.

Over time, I have worked to develop a safe, gentle, and effective way for people to heal from trauma. It works by understanding that trauma is primarily *physiological*. Trauma is something that happens initially to our bodies and our instincts. Only then do its effects spread to our minds, emotions, and spirits.

MOVING OUT OF IMMOBILITY

The question is: how can humans become unstuck from immobility? Moving out of this frozen state can be a fiercely energetic experience. Without a rational brain, animals in the wild don't give it a second thought—they simply do it. When humans begin to move out of the immobility response, however, we are often frightened by the intensity of our own energy and latent aggression, and we brace ourselves against the power of the sensations. This bracing prevents the complete discharge of energy necessary to restore normal functioning. Un-discharged energy is stored in the nervous system, setting the stage for the formation of the symptoms of trauma, which we discussed in the previous chapter. So, how do we get unstuck? How do we release this frozen energy so that we can move from trauma, which is fixity, to flow?

That is precisely what you are about to learn in my Twelve-Phase Healing Trauma Program.

A GENTLE, GRADUAL APPROACH TO HEALING TRAUMA

In the twelve phases introduced in the next chapter, and available on the CD that accompanies this book, you'll learn how to release yourself from the bondage of unresolved traumas from your past.

When we can discharge our residual survival energy, we feel less threatened and overwhelmed by life. We are no longer frozen in fear. While we are frozen, any movement is frightening, chaotic. As we move from fixity to flow, we begin to experience a sense of coherency. We begin to feel reconnected to life. We feel more peaceful, at home with others, the world, and ourselves. We are no longer trapped by events in our past, some of which we may not even remember.

This brings up a very important fact: that is, you don't have to consciously remember an event to heal from it. Visiting one's trauma is quite different from reliving it. Because trauma happens primarily on an instinctive level, the memories we have of overwhelming events are stored as fragmentary experiences in our bodies, not in the rational parts of our brains.

When we are able to access our "body memories" through the felt sense, then we can begin to discharge the instinctive survival energy that we did not have a chance to use at the time of an event.

Regardless of what your particular situation is, you can learn to discharge and transform this energy. The discharge can be dramatic and visible, or subtle and quiet. It can be an intense shivering or the slightest sense of inner trembling; or it may be a changing of temperature between hot and cold, between warmth and coolness. Afterwards, you might notice that things fall into place a little easier, or that you're calmer and more relaxed. Perhaps things that once upset you won't seem to bother you as much, and you are significantly less critical of yourself. Or, you might experience a subtle deepening of your sense of well-being.

It's also entirely possible that the change may be more profound. Chronic pain may disappear. You might be able to do things that you've never before attempted. Your relationships with loved ones and others might become freer and easier. You might experience a surge in your feelings of passion and personal power. When trauma is healed, shift happens.

This approach to trauma is not psychotherapy, nor does it replace psychotherapy. I often worked with people who are referred to me by their therapists. Just as often, people who come to me are not involved in psychotherapy. Many of them have been in automobile or other types of accidents, and are suffering from short- or long-term chronic pain.

Psychotherapy can be an important tool for many trauma sufferers. Sometimes, professional help is necessary, and you may choose to share this book with your therapist, social worker, doctor, or any other professional with whom you might be working.

But I want to emphasize that, by using the techniques presented in this integrated book/CD, many of you will be able to help each other, your children, family and friends, both prevent and resolve your own traumas. I wish you the best of luck in your personal healing journey.

CHAPTER
FOUR

Twelve-Phase Healing Trauma Program: A Guide to the Audio Exercises

AFTER READING THE BOOK to this point, you can begin working with the exercises. There are two more chapters that follow the exercises, one that provides special insights into sexual trauma, and one that looks at the spiritual portals that open to you as you work on resolving and healing your trauma. There is also an additional section on "trauma first aid" for adults and children, which would be best read after doing the exercises. However, if you prefer to read the text first, the exercises will still be effective. In addition, a condensed version of some of the exercises is presented in the text. You can, if you want, also do them this way if it is helpful to you.

Initially, it's important to do the phases in the order in which I've presented them. Each phase can contain one or more exercises. I suggest working with Phase 1, then taking a day or two to observe your responses and possible changes as a result. Then you can proceed to Phase 2. Make sure you give each phase in turn a day or two to reveal its effects before moving on to the following one.

Remember, there's no need to rush. You don't need to stop doing each exercise once the audio presentation is done. In fact, I encourage you to continue working on your own after each track ends.

Ultimately, all of the phases will help you get reacquainted with feelings and sensations in your own body. People who have experienced trauma are often cut off from their bodies, so these exercises may seem to open up a whole new world for you. This process takes time. Even if you understand and think you "get" the exercises, your body may need some time to integrate and incorporate the lessons. Learning the language of the body is much like learning a foreign language. The language of the body has its own grammar and syntax and idioms, and there's no way to learn it in just one day.

As you move through the phases, you can continue to revisit and practice earlier exercises as often as you wish. For example, Phase I, which helps you find your body boundaries, can be very useful to practice on a regular basis. You can return to this phase either by listening to the first audio track again, or simply by applying the techniques in other situations—while standing in line at the grocery store, for example.

After a week and a half to two weeks, you will likely have completed the twelve phases in order. (If it takes you longer, that's okay, too.) At that point, it's up to you to decide which phases to do again and how often to do them.

You may find that a particular exercise—perhaps one that didn't have a strong impact on you he first time you did it—will take on greater meaning as you revisit it. Sometimes techniques learned in the later phases will give you new insights into earlier phases.

If you feel drawn to practice certain exercises on a regular basis, go ahead and do so. The first and last phases are particularly helpful for grounding, and can be used successfully whenever you feel overwhelmed or off-center.

You should try to really bring these exercises into your life until you've internalized these skills and can practice them in different contexts. The body awareness these twelve phases help cultivate does more than simply aid us in recovering from unresolved trauma. Body awareness is something we want to cultivate and make an intrinsic part of our lives, because living in a body-aware way gives us a sense of aliveness and purpose in all aspects of life. When we're disconnected from the body, we can't be fully present. A meaningful life depends upon a sense of aliveness and presence, both of which spring from intimate contact with internal body states. As Willhelm Reich, M.D., said, "Love, work, and understanding should be the wellsprings of our life. They should also govern it."

GETTING RESULTS

Many people ask me how long it will take to get results from these exercises. The answer is, it depends. Many people begin to feel the benefits of these practices almost immediately, but the results will differ for different people, depending on the type and amount of trauma you've suffered. Don't be discouraged if you don't feel changes immediately, because this is also common. Remember, trauma robs us of our body sense. These exercises are a way of reconnecting with the body, but for some people being in the body is so uncomfortable and fraught with difficult feelings that it can take some time to reestablish that connection and befriend your body.

If you work with these exercises over time, many traumas can move towards resolution. If the traumas in your past were particularly overwhelming, it's possible that future events can cause certain symptoms to reappear, even if the stuck energy of this past trauma was discharged though the use of these techniques.

I've worked with people who were able to resolve trauma and get rid of symptoms, only to have symptoms reappear when a new trauma occurs. However, I've also found that, as a result of consistent work with these exercises, people are able to develop greater resiliency, and are more prepared to work through trauma symptoms should they resurface. These body-based exercises can actually help make you even stronger than you were before your initial trauma occurred.

GO EASY ON YOURSELF

If at any time either the subject being discussed or the exercises seem disturbing, *stop and let things settle.* Sit with your experience and see what unfolds. As you listen, keep a portion of your attention on your responses to the information you are receiving. You might want to take a "break," to take a short walk and come back to it later. Remember, *body sensations, rather than intense emotion, are the key to healing trauma.*

Be aware of any emotional reaction swelling up inside you, and of how your body is experiencing these emotions in the form of sensations and thoughts. Some things to watch for are emotions that feel too intense to manage—rage, terror, profound helplessness—or getting flooded with disturbing images or perhaps having the compulsion to carry out some potentially dangerous fantasy.

In cases like these, you may need to enlist competent professional help. *This is important. Please seriously consider seeking the assistance of a professionally trained therapist.* You can also find a list of practitioners trained in working with this approach to trauma at the web site: www.traumahealing.com.

FIND A SAFE PLACE

NOTE: Only do these body awareness exercises when you are in a safe place, possibly with a spouse or a friend. Do not attempt them while driving or while doing anything else that requires your attention.

This work is often best done in the presence of another person. The reason for this is that human beings do not feel completely safe when alone, especially when we need to focus our attention inside ourselves. The presence of another allows us to feel safe so that we may better make this heroic inner journey.

THE TWELVE-PHASE HEALING TRAUMA PROGRAM

FIRST GROUP: PREPARATORY PHASES

The first three phases work with some fundamental resources that are lost or damaged in trauma, and help you begin to repair them. Before trauma, you are not overwhelmed by your feelings. After trauma, feelings can be completely overwhelming.

When you have been traumatized, you're often unable to feel your own physical boundaries, because of disconnection from your body. This can have an impact in other areas of life, such as setting boundaries in relationships, because it's impossible to set limits if you have no sense of your own boundaries. Rebuilding connection is really the key to all of these exercises, because trauma is about loss of connection, first to the body and self, and second to others and the environment.

Phase 1 — Safety and Containment Exercises: Finding Your Body Boundaries
Preparation

The body is the container of *all* of our sensation and feelings. It is also the boundary separating us from our environment and from others. This boundary gets ruptured in trauma so that we often feel raw and unprotected. Skin is our first line of defense. Then our muscles give us the sense of an ego-boundary between self and other. This phase is designed to help repair that rupture so that you can feel safer and more intact.

To begin the containment exercises that constitute Phase I, find a comfortable place to sit. I invite you to notice a couple of things. First, notice how the back of the chair supports your spine and how the base of the chair supports your bottom. If the chair has arms, notice how it feels to have your arms' weight supported, also.

Next, take enough time so that you feel that support in a direct physical way in order to literally feel the back of the chair straightening your spine. When you have that sense, it may be strong and definite, or it may rather be vague. If it's vague at first, don't worry about it. As you do these exercises over and over again, you will find that you get increasing awareness each time. The main idea, as you practice, is to begin to feel your skin and your muscles as boundaries holding and containing your sensations and feelings.

In Chapter 2, we learned about the symptoms of dissociation and denial so common in trauma. In dissociation, we vacate our bodies in some way or another. We can experience anything from a little spaciness all the way to feeling completely disconnected, numb, fragmented, or unreal. In order to heal trauma, we must learn how to safely come back into our bodies by experiencing them as a container for our feelings. We will begin with some simple restorative exercises.

LISTEN TO TRACK ONE
Safety and Containment Exercises:
Finding Your Body Boundaries

Practice
NOTE: In order to perform some portions of these exercises, you'll need to have available a massaging showerhead and a ball of string or yarn. If you don't have a showerhead, proceed with the exercises and go back to the shower exercise once you've purchased the showerhead.

Tapping exercise. To begin, gently tap the palm of your left hand with the fingers of your right hand. Do this as many times as you need to get a sense of that part of your body. Then, stop tapping and take the time to notice the sensation in the palm of your hand. What do you feel? Do you feel tingly? Do you feel a vibration? Do you feel numb? Hot or cold? Just take a few moments to notice whatever you feel.

Now, look at your hand and say, "This is my hand, my hand belongs to me, my hand is a part of me." (You can use any words that seem right to help you get the idea of *ownership* of each part of yourself as belonging to a greater whole.)

Next, turn your hand over and begin tapping on the back of your hand. Again, notice any sensation. Follow the sensation for a moment, noticing how it changes. Use whatever words feel most appropriate to convey a sense of ownership.

Continue leading yourself through every part of your body: lower and upper arms, feet, calves, thighs, abdomen, upper torso, buttocks, back, neck, face, and head. Take as much time as necessary to complete this portion of the exercise. You may pause the CD and continue on your own for as long as feels comfortable before moving on to the next portion.

This initial skin boundary exercise may take as much as an hour. What's important is that you develop an ability to pace yourself and recognize your *own* window of tolerance, gently increasing your comfort zone over time.

Shower exercise. Now, let's do another version of working with your skin boundary. If you choose to try this one, you will need to purchase an inexpensive pulsing showerhead, if you don't already have one. Adjust the shower to a comfortable temperature and a comfortable level of intensity. Put your hand up to the shower, feel the pulsing on your hand and again say, "This is the palm of my hand; I feel the palm of my hand. It belongs to me; it's part of my body."

Again, use the particular wording that feels right to you. Then turn the back of your hand to the water and repeat the exercise. Do this with as many parts of your body as you want to do at that time. In other words, the procedure is exactly the same as in the previous exercise, only you're using the pulsating water for contact instead of tapping.

String boundary exercise. Now take a ball of yarn or string and seat yourself comfortably on the floor. Focus on the front, sides, and back of your body, paying attention to where you feel your own personal boundary is. In other words, if someone were to come closer than this boundary, you might begin to feel uncomfortable. Use the yarn or string to mark out what you feel is your personal boundary. If you are with someone, you can practice saying to that person something like, "These are my boundaries; you may only come in, beyond them, if I invite you in."

Muscle exercise. Now that you've gotten some sense of your skin boundary and the container it provides for you, we'll focus on an even more solid container: the deeper boundary of your muscles. To begin, take your right hand and put it on the side of your left upper arm. Squeeze the muscle gently but firmly so that you can really feel the density and shape of your muscle. Again say something like, "This is my muscle. This is part of me. This is a deeper container for my feelings and my sensations."

Next, you might move your awareness to your shoulders, squeezing them a few times, feeling the tension build as you squeeze and feeling the release as you let it go. Again find your own rhythm of squeezing each muscle and letting it go.

When you first try this exercise, you may need to apply more pressure to get the feeling, but the idea is to use just enough pressure to get a sense of your muscle. So, as you feel and squeeze those parts of your body, you are beginning to actually feel the container and the boundary of your feelings.

Remember to take as much time as you need to go over each part of your body in order to reacquaint yourself with it and how it is connected with every other part.

As we did in the skin tapping exercise, it may be beneficial to say to yourself the affirmations that we have gone over for each part of your body. Make your statements slowly and compassionately as you feel each muscle and how it's connected to your whole body. You might even find it helpful to mention its function as you squeeze. For example, you might say, "This is my calf muscle; it helps me stand my ground; it helps me run quickly."

Although a considerable amount of change may be experienced doing these exercises just one time, it is more likely that you will get the most benefit by repeating these exercises, progressing with more awareness and comfort over time. It will also help to do them in conjunction with the other exercises in this learning program.

In doing these exercises and building a sense of your body as your container, you will find a greater capacity to befriend some of the uncomfortable sensations and feelings you may have previously disconnected.

Phase 2 — Grounding and Centering

Preparation

Trauma disconnects people from their bodies. In love, we are "swept off our feet." In trauma, our legs are pulled out from under us. Grounding and centering, as you shall see, reconnects you directly with resources naturally available in your own body. It is important to reestablish your relationship to both the ground and to your body's center of gravity, the place where action and feeling originate. These functions are compromised in trauma. In trauma, people lose their ground, so an important part of healing is learning to reestablish ground. As you ground and center yourself before each of the exercises in this program, it will help you create a feeling of safety, a sense that you cannot so easily be knocked off balance by your emotions, sensations, or thoughts.

You'll need a chair to complete one of the exercises in this phase. Another exercise calls for an animal friend. If you have a pet, make sure the animal is nearby. If you don't have a pet, you might borrow a friend's pet—one which you are comfortable with—for this purpose. It's also okay to go ahead and skip that one exercise.

Practice

To begin, stand and simply feel your feet on the ground. Notice the springiness and stiffness in your legs. Feel the way your feet contact the ground, almost like suction cups. With your feet firmly planted, sway slowly from the ankles, first from side to side, and then forward and backward. This will help you locate your center of gravity, in the upper pelvic area. Place your hands on your lower belly and sense your center of gravity. It may be helpful to continue swaying gently while doing this.

Chair exercise. Now sit in a chair with your feet on the ground or the floor. (It does not matter if you are twenty stories up). Place your hands on your lower belly and sense the energy coming up from the ground and into that area through your feet and legs.

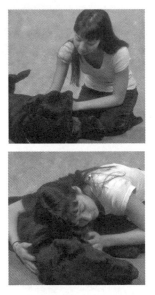

Animal exercise. Another way to help ground yourself is to work with an animal. Animals are completely natural, grounded, and instinctual. Even a poodle raised in the city still retains its instincts. Sometimes you can get a sense of groundedness simply by watching animals—for example, by watching a cat and noticing how completely in rhythm and in the body the animal is. Frequently, traumatized people have pets for exactly that reason.

You may also wish to work more closely with an animal, by placing your hands on its body or your head upon its chest. Notice the calmness in the animal. Listen to its heartbeat and feel its breathing. Feel yourself settle in to the animal's own natural rhythms. You may try this for as long as feels comfortable for both you and the animal. As little as a few minutes may have a noticeable effect.

Phase 3 — Building Resources

Preparation

Everybody has resources. It can also be said that every *body* has resources. What are resources and where do they come from? Resources can be anything or anyone that supports and nurtures a sense of physical, emotional, mental, and spiritual well-being. They can be obvious or hidden. They can be active or forgotten. They can be external, internal, or both. Simple examples of external resources might be: nature, friends, family, animals, athletics, dance, music, and other expressive arts. Examples of internal resources might be: strength, agility, intelligence, a spiritual practice, inherent talents, instinctual wisdom, and a resilient nervous system.

When a person has been traumatized, instinctive resources for successful protection and self-defense have been overwhelmed in part or in whole. Resources can be lost or forgotten after even one traumatizing event. If trauma began during the formative years of infancy and early childhood, few resources may have been available from the beginning.

During this resource-building exercise, you will recover some of your body's innate resources and perhaps even discover new ones.

For this exercise, you'll need paper and pen.

Practice

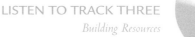

LISTEN TO TRACK THREE
Building Resources

Take a piece of paper. Or you can use a page from your journal, if you have one. Divide your page vertically in half so that you have two columns. In one column, begin a list of your external resources; in the other column, list your internal resources.

Over time, you can continue to add to each list. If you find that you are lacking resources you wish you had, such as people and physical exercise, you might decide to join a Tai Chi class or find a walking buddy to help you move out of isolation into both more activity and connectedness.

As we move into the second group of exercises (Tracking), you will discover how to more fully embody the resources from your lists that bring you comfort and safety.

If you have difficulty beginning your list, take some time to recall what got you through your trauma. How did you cope? What helped you the most to get to the place you are now? What inner strengths did you bring to bear in your struggle to go on with life? If you suffered early abuse, who or what helped you to survive your childhood trauma? Take a few moments to imagine or feel possible resources, even if they seem distant, vague, or weak. Little by little, you will notice emergent resources that have been lost, find new ones, and strengthen those that are weak.

SECOND GROUP: TRACKING SKILLS

In the first group of phases, you learned to contain sensations and feelings, restore a sense of center, and begin to restore your body boundaries. After the three phases, you will begin to feel less betrayed and more supported by your body.

In the next three phases, you'll begin to learn the language of inner bodily experiences. Perhaps your body has felt frozen or paralyzed by fear, or collapsed in shame or helplessness. During these next phases, you'll be able to feel where you've collapsed, where the body is tensed or constricted, and begin to normalize that sensation through feeling and movement.

These phases are tools to feel into your body, sense what parts of the body have too much or not enough energy, and begin to create conduits for stuck energy to flow. When you find the places you're stuck, you're ready to become unstuck, because each of these places is a movement and energy ready to be continued and completed.

Phase 4 — From "Felt Sense" to Tracking Specific Sensations
Preparation

Before beginning the exercises in this section, it's important that you fully understand the key concept of *felt sense.* According to Eugene Gendlin, the author of the seminal book *Focusing,* who has coined the term *felt sense:* "A felt sense is not a mental experience but a physical one. *Physical.* A bodily awareness of a situation or person or event. An internal aura that encompasses everything you feel and know about the given subject at a given time."

The felt sense can be said to be the medium through which we experience the totality of sensation. Every event can be experienced both as individual parts and as a unified whole. To harness the instincts necessary to heal trauma, we must be able to identify and employ the indicators of trauma that are made available to us through the felt sense.

Being consciously aware of your body and its sensations makes any experience more intense. It is important to recognize that the experience of comfort, for example, comes from your felt sense of comfort and not from the chair, the sofa, or whatever surface you are sitting on. As a visit to any furniture store will soon reveal, you can't know that a chair is comfortable until you sit on it and get a bodily sense of what it feels like.

The felt sense blends together most of the information that forms your experience. Even when you are not consciously aware of it, the felt sense is telling you where you are and how you feel at any given moment. It is relaying the overall experience of the organism, rather than interpreting what is happening from the standpoint of the individual parts. Perhaps the best way to describe the felt sense is to say that it is the experience of being in a living body that understands the nuances of its environment by way of its responses to that environment.

In many ways, the felt sense is like a stream moving through an ever-changing landscape. It alters its character in resonance with its surroundings. When the land is rugged and steep, the stream moves with vigor and energy, swirling and bubbling as it crashes over rocks and debris. Out on the plains, the stream meanders so slowly that one might wonder whether it is moving at all. In the same way, once the setting has been interpreted and defined by the felt sense, we blend into whatever conditions we find ourselves placed in. Like the stream, this amazing sense shapes itself to those environments.

The physical (external) senses of sight, sound, smell, touch, and taste are elements that contribute only a portion of the information that builds the foundation for the felt sense. Other important data are derived from our body's internal awareness—the positions it takes, the tensions it has, the movements it makes, its temperature, etc. The felt sense can be influenced, even changed by our thought. Yet it's not a thought; rather, it's something we feel.

Emotions contribute to the felt sense, but they play a less important role than most people believe. Emotions such as sorrow, anger, fear, disgust, and joy are intense and direct. There are a limited variety of these types of feelings, and they are easily recognized and named. This is not so with the felt sense.

The felt sense encompasses a complex array of ever-shifting nuances. The feelings we experience are typically much more subtle, complex, and intricate than what we can convey in language.

As you read the following phrases, imagine how much more you might feel, experiencing these things, than can possibly be expressed in words:

- Looking at a mountain peak bathed in an alpine glow
- Seeing a blue summer sky dotted with soft white clouds

- Going to a ball game and dripping mustard on your shirt
- Feeling the ocean spray as the surf crashes onto rock and cliff
- Touching an opening rose or a blade of grass topped with a drop of morning dew
- Listening to a Brahms concerto
- Watching a group of brightly dressed children singing ethnic folk songs
- Walking along a country road
- Enjoying conversation with a friend

You can imagine going through a day without emotion, but to live in the absence of the felt sense is not just unthinkable; it is impossible. To live without the felt sense violates the most basic experience of being alive.

The felt sense is sometimes vague, often complex, and ever-changing. It moves, shifts, and transforms constantly. It can vary in intensity and clarity, enabling us to shift our perceptions. It does this by giving us the process as well as what is needed for change. Through the felt sense we are able to move, to acquire new information, to interrelate with one another and, ultimately, to know who we are. It is so integral to our experience of being human that we take it for granted, sometimes to the point of not even realizing that it exists until we deliberately attend to it. To the degree that you experience the felt sense as ever-shifting and are able to embrace this constant flow, then you will be moving out of trauma into life.

Describing and Tracking Sensation. Before you begin working with the exercises on Track Four, I'd like you give some thought to the words that you use to describe how you feel. This process will help you better acquaint yourself with identifying and describing your physical sensations.

When someone asks you how you're doing, you may typically answer in a vague way, such as, "okay" or "not so good."

But try asking yourself, "What sensation *in my body* tells me that I'm feeling okay?" You may well get some more information: "My head feels heavy. My left shoulder is tingly. And my hand is warm."

Fear might be experienced as a rapid heartbeat or a knot in the gut. You see how much more specific that description is, how much more connected to your body? This may feel like a different language to you at first, but with practice, it will become easier.

Below is a list of terms you may find helpful to get you started with describing your bodily sensations:

Dense	Thick	Flowing
Breathless	Fluttery	Nervous
Queasy	Expanded	Floating
Heavy	Tingly	Electric
Fluid	Numb	Wooden
Dizzy	Full	Congested
Spacey	Trembly	Twitchy
Tight	Hot	Bubbly
Achy	Wobbly	Calm
Suffocating	Buzzy	Energized
Tremulous	Constricted	Warm
Knotted	Icy	Light
Blocked	Hollow	Cold
Disconnected	Sweaty	Streaming

The way that you distinguish a sensation from an emotion and from a thought is by being able to locate it in your body and experience it in a direct physical way. For example, if you're experiencing anxiety, the next question to ask would be: "When I feel anxious, how do I know that I am feeling anxious?" In other words, *where* in your body do you feel it, and exactly what is the physical sensation? Is it tightness? Is it constriction? Is it a knot? Or, is it a fluttery feeling? Is it your heart palpitating? What is your breathing like? Are there butterflies in your stomach? All of these sensations might be called "anxiety." The trick in dealing with and finding a sensation is to realize that it has to have a location in the body. It can have a size. It frequently has a shape. And it has a specific physical quality, such as tightness, spaciousness, constriction, heat, cold, vibration, or tingling.

Now you're ready to proceed with Phase 4.

Practice

NOTE: for the following exercise, you'll need an object (or even a person—or image of them) that is special to you. This object will serve as the focus of the exercise.

LISTEN TO TRACK FOUR
From "Felt Sense" to Tracking Specific Sensations

When we have been traumatized, the body doesn't feel like a safe place. It feels like a dangerous place. This exercise is designed to help you discover your own pacing and inner rhythms, and to trust in your own innate capacity to regulate and to heal. It will help you begin to find islands of relative safety or ease within your body.

Find a comfortable place to sit, either in a chair or on the floor. I prefer that you start by sitting rather than lying down, because sometimes when you lie down, the sensations and feeling can come up more quickly and be more difficult. And, please, never try this exercise while driving.

As you practice, slow down or stop altogether if the sensations begin to get too intense. Remember that your tolerance will build gradually, as you continue with all of these exercises.

Begin by bringing into your space something that gives you sense of comfort or is special to you. It could be a stone, a crystal, a flower, a pet, a favorite picture or photograph. It could even be a trusted friend you want simply to sit with you in quiet support.

Now tune in to the sensations your body is experiencing. Feel how the chair or floor holds your weight. Notice your clothing on your skin, and begin to place your awareness on the muscles underneath your skin as well. Notice how your feet are grounded, through the floor and the foundation and down into the earth. Try to feel this sense of groundedness with your whole body.

Now gaze at your object of safety, and slowly move your attention back and forth between your body and the object in front of you. If, for example, you have a stone in front of you, look at the stone with a sense of your bodily experiences in the background. Then shift your awareness so that the image in front of you recedes and you become more aware of your bodily experience.

You might ask yourself if your object makes you feel more solid, centered, or grounded. Where in your body do you feel that sense, and what is the physical sensation? Continue for several minutes to shift back and forth, at your own rhythm, between the object and the sensations in your body.

Now allow your focus to shift to an inner sense of where the comfort is experienced in your body, and take some time to explore the nuances of this sensation. Where does the sense of comfort begin? Perhaps you sense tense muscles beginning to let go, or a sense of spaciousness around your heart, or warmth in your belly. Perhaps you were feeling anxious initially, and this feeling has changed in some small way.

Observe these sensations and follow these changes. It might not feel like much is happening at first. Conversely, it might feel like too much is happening. You can adjust your experience to fit your need by shifting focus between your sensations and the comfortable object or image that you chose as resource. Remember that you are in control.

Conflict-free exercise. Now that you feel comfortable shifting between the outer object and your inner bodily sensations, I'd like to introduce the next stage of this exercise. I would like for you to recollect a time in the past few days when you felt most like yourself. Perhaps at that moment you felt closer to your true self, or to the self you want to be. Perhaps you felt more pleasure or less anxiety than usual.

As you think of that time, I want to you to notice what your bodily experience is, again without judging it. Simply notice it. Just shift back and forth rhythmically, like a pendulum, between your image or memory of that event and the current sensations in your body.

Next, think about something that happened in the last week or two, when again you felt the most like yourself. Again, simply shift your awareness back and forth between the remembrance or the mental picture of that moment and your current bodily experience, whatever it may be. Stay with this process for a few minutes, shifting your focus back and forth between the picture or remembrance and your bodily sensations, simply noticing the process without judgment.

Next, moving a little further backwards in time, I want you to think of a situation in the last month or so when you felt most like yourself, the self you want to be. As you think of that time, holding the image in your mind's eye, again take time to shift back and forth between the image and your bodily sensations. Pendulate back and forth, feeling the rhythm of your awareness shifting from the remembrance to the sensation, from the sensation to the remembrance. Allow the sensation to grow, so that you're aware of your entire body.

Now, slowly begin to think about opening your eyes and coming back into the room. When you're ready, slowly open your eyes and gaze at the special object in front of you. Simply look at that object, begin to shift back and forth between your observation of the object outside and your internal experience, again just feeling the rhythm of this pendulation in your body. As you are coming back out into the world, you might want to incorporate elements of the body boundaries exercise, squeezing your muscles with your hands, or tapping gently on different parts of your body.

Phase 5 — Tracking Activation: Sensations, Images, Thoughts, and Emotions
Preparation

If you noticed yourself trying to figure it out or attach some kind of significance to the sensations you tracked in the previous phase, try the following technique as you continue to practice tracking skills in Phase 5. If a thought arises and activates you in an unpleasant way, say to yourself, "I just had a thought. What do I begin to notice in my body now?"

By bringing yourself back to your body, you can track the effect of that thought on your bodily sensations. When you're not able to recognize the thought as a thought, the unpleasant sensations the thought evokes may increase until you are feeling fear, anxiety, or panic. In other words, you are bringing yourself back to your body, and you can even notice the thought that you are having, but you notice that it's a thought. If you tighten up without noticing the thought that caused the tightening, your response tends to be more catastrophic, leading you to believe that something bad is going to happen. And then, all of a sudden, the tightness increases and "out of the blue" you are feeling fear, anxiety, or even panic.

With closer examination, you can see that the negative thought and the tightness in the body mutually reinforced one another to actually generate the states of fear or panic. By being aware of this interaction, you'll be better able simply to track the bodily sensations arising from thought without being at their mercy.

Follow this same procedure with any images that may arise as you practice the next phase. These images may be visual, auditory (sound or voice), gustatory (taste), olfactory (smell), or tactile (touch). Remember to ask, "When I have an image of _____, what sensation do I notice in my body?"

A key in moving through trauma is learning to separate out the sensations, thoughts, images, and emotions that may cause arousal. When you are able to note and track sensations as they change, instead of being stuck in habitual traumatic patterning, then thoughts and images that used to cause strong reactions will begin to lose their hold on you.

The next phase will take the form of guided imagery that may arouse some strong emotions in you. Remember, if at any time you feel overwhelmed, simply stop the exercise and come back to it later or even after a couple of days.

Practice

NOTE: This exercise must be performed in conjunction with the audio track. Please refer to Track Five for instructions.

LISTEN TO TRACK FIVE

Tracking Activation: Sensations, Images, Thoughts, and Emotions

Phase 6 — Pendulation: Tracking Your Rhythms of Expansion and Contraction
Preparation

When we enter a new situation, we're activated to focus our attention on this new event. However, traumatized people tend to be riveted on their traumas; new situations are connected to—and constricted by—that past event. The key to dissolving this constriction is simply learning to stay with the sensation until it begins to change.

When you contact that stuck sensation, it *will* begin to change, simply because that's the nature of all sensation. However, when you come in contact with that constriction for the first time, it can often give rise to fear. Indeed, the sensation is likely to get worse before it gets better because, for the first time, you're experiencing it directly. As you stay with it, it may continue to get worse, then better, in a cycle of expansion and contraction. What's important to realize is that you can *pendulate*—swing back and forth—between these sensations of expansion and contraction. And this means that you're no longer stuck!

As you work with the next exercise, you might try a vocalization that I find helps the stuckness dissolve more quickly. Take a deep breath, and vocalize the sound voooooo (or *vuuuuuuu*) for your full out-breath. Then, when it's ready, allow a new breath to come in fully as it wants. Continue with the vocalization until you feel more comfortable pendulating between contraction and expansion.

Once you learn to pendulate successfully, you'll discover that your seemingly infinite emotional pain begins to feel manageable and finite. This shift allows your attention to move from dread and helplessness to curiosity and exploration. Your task is simply learning to observe what is going on inside you, without being carried away by over-stimulation or losing interest out of "boredom."

In the following exercises, I ask you not to try to interpret, analyze, or explain what is happening. Just experience and note it. It is unnecessary to dredge up memories, emotions, insights, or anything else for that matter. If they come, that's fine. But it is more important to observe them without interpretation or emotional attachment. Look at them; then let them go. Take it as it comes. This is the best way to learn the language of your felt sense. It is like sitting on the banks of a stream, watching the water flow by.

Practice

LISTEN TO TRACK SIX
*Pendulation: Tracking Your Rhythms
of Expansion and Contraction*

Now, I want you to recall an experience in which you felt mildly uncomfortable. Imagine you are in your car, on your way home from shopping or work. You are feeling calm, but are looking forward to getting home. You notice that the cars in front of you are slowing down. You put on the brakes, and slowly come to a stop. You are in a traffic jam. You can't see the cause of the jam, because it's too far away. Now, I want you to notice what you are experiencing in your felt sense. If you're feeling the usual irritation, etc. of being stuck in a traffic jam, just sit with it a while and notice what your body is experiencing. In other words, pay attention to how and where your body feels irritated. Then just focus on the physical sensation until it begins to shift; notice these rhythms of expansion and contraction.

If you feel overwhelmed or deeply disturbed during any part of this exercise on the CD, please stop the exercise and return to it again at a later time. The exercise may be too activating for some people. If this is true for you, I suggest you stop and focus on a pleasant experience you had recently, or just sit or take a short walk and allow yourself to "normalize."

THIRD GROUP: DISCHARGING ACTIVATION

In this third group of exercises, you'll begin to work with the two basic survival responses, the fight response and the flight response. With the tracking skills presented in the previous group of exercises, you've learned that there are places in the body where we're stuck as a result of incomplete responses to our need to fight or escape. When we have these incomplete responses, we tend to collapse. In other words, if fight is not an option and flight is not an option, then the default option in the nervous system and body is paralysis and collapse. This is simply how we're wired for survival.

By being able to contact both our natural aggression and our flight response, we can create new channels for this compressed and collapsed energy to complete its movement and course of action. When this stuck energy is restored to the whole organism, we can begin to live more fully—to create, accomplish, communicate, collaborate, and share. Instead of being engaged merely in survival, we can then come back to our balanced place, where we're basically social animals. The fear and paralysis and dread drop away, and we come back into the present, because we have access to all of the energy previously bound up in our freezing and immobility, in our incomplete fight and flight responses.

Phase 7 — Fight Response: Natural Aggression versus Violence
Preparation

Aggression is an innate natural resource that protects us when we are threatened. It is also the force that mobilizes us to action and propels us towards our desires and goals in life. When people have been traumatized, they are stuck in paralysis—the immobility reaction or abrupt explosions of rage. Because of this, they lack the healthy aggression that they need to carry out their lives effectively.

Nature has designed us, like most other animals, to access aggression when we need to defend ourselves, and when we begin to emerge from immobility. This only makes sense, because if the predator is still in the area, counter-attack may be all that we have for defending our lives. Traumatized people, generally, have become fearful of their own aggression. Hence, when they begin to emerge from immobility (with its inherent aggression), they suppress this life-saving aggressive response. This suppression has the consequence of throwing them back into paralysis. Thus, with their aggression aborted, they remain fearful of re-engaging in life.

Often, traumatized people either feel nothing or they feel rage, and often the rage is expressed in inappropriate ways. By beginning to get a sense of what healthy aggression feels like, the extremes of numbness and rage can begin to give way to a healthier middle ground. The following exercises help establish feelings of healthy aggression and empowerment. Practicing in this way creates a positive channel for emotions that might surface. As with all the exercises, do these after you are centered and grounded.

The exercises in Phase 7 require two people. Ask a trusted friend or family member to work with you.

Practice

Push hands exercise. This technique requires two people: the *pusher* and the *pushee*. Place the palm

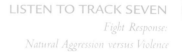

LISTEN TO TRACK SEVEN
Fight Response:
Natural Aggression versus Violence

of one hand comfortably against the palm of your partner's hand. If you are the pusher, begin to feel strength and force arising from your center. Start slowly exerting pressure on the pushee. Push as far as you like, while keeping your balance.

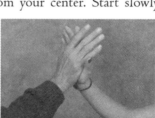

The pushee's job is simply to be there and to provide the resistance necessary to meet the pressure by mirroring the pusher's strength. Some eye contact is beneficial, but too much can be overwhelming.

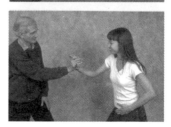

Take turns playing the role of the pusher and the pushee. When you are the pushee, if you sense that the pusher is collapsing or backing off, reduce eye contact until you feel the pusher has regained his or her strength. Decrease resis-

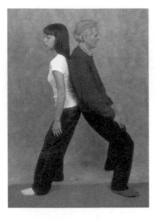

tance slightly from time to time to determine if the pusher is maintaining his or her balance.

Back pushing exercise. Start with your back against your partner's back while maintaining the feeling of being grounded. Feel the inner support in your upper and lower back. If you experience some gentle shaking and trembling while sinking into this support, just allow it to happen. Take all the time you need. Then slowly begin to push. As in the first exercise, the pusher determines the amount of force while the pushee offers matching resistance. Feel the power coming from your legs and center.

Take turns being both the pusher and the pushee.

Phase 8 — Flight Response: Natural Escape versus Anxiety

Preparation

When we have been traumatized, it's often because we found ourselves in a situation from which we couldn't escape. Our natural flight response was thwarted or overwhelmed. This leads to a feeling of being stuck and frightened—a pervasive feeling for traumatized people in many different areas of life.

By the same token, if in the past you froze when you were threatened, in all likelihood you'll freeze again in the future when confronted with an activating situation such as an argument or intimate encounter. This sense of immobility can lead to a pervasive dread of the future. On the other hand, if you feel confident that you can escape when threatened, that feeling of dread begins to dissolve. You no longer feel overwhelmed. This exercise is designed to give you a sense of your ability to escape when necessary.

Practice

Sit in a comfortable chair with a sturdy foam pillow under your feet, and ground yourself. Close
your eyes and imagine that a fierce baboon is chasing
you. Feel the strength in your legs as you make running
movements on the pillow. Remain mindful of your legs
and body as you do this. Run until you reach a safe place
on top of a large boulder. You have escaped. The baboon
loses interest and wanders away. Sit on the warm rock
and allow yourself to settle. Notice your breathing and
heartbeat. If you begin to shake and tremble, simply
allow it to happen. You can also imagine other situations—present or past—where you wanted to run and
felt that, in some way, you were prevented. When you

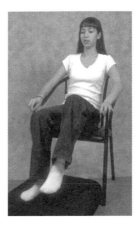

LISTEN TO TRACK EIGHT

*Flight Response: Natural Escape
versus Anxiety*

have that image you can again experience your running response. I suggest, though,
that before you do this you think about the safe place (or person) that you would
want to run to. Again, it is good to have someone whom you trust to sit in the
room with you.

Phase 9 — Strength and Resiliency versus Collapse and Defeat

Preparation

The feeling of collapse that traumatized people often experience in the face of life
situations can be seen as an incomplete response to threat. By learning to complete
this collapse response by going into, and out of, it fully, you can begin to regain
a sense of strength and resiliency in any challenging situation. This completed
response makes it all but impossible to remain in the depressed state associated with
the sensation of collapse.

Practice

When we've been overwhelmed or humiliated, our bodies tend to collapse. Our shoulders go forward, our eyes avert downwards, and we collapse around the area of our diaphragm into our abdomen. Now, I want you to just feel in your body what it feels like to experience that sense of collapse. If you wish, you can think of a time when you felt defeated or shamed in some way. Just use that image, and feel how your body collapses.

Now, rather than fight the collapse, what I want you to do is allow your body, a little bit at a time, to fall further into the collapse, staying mindful all the time. Then, when it feels like you've reached an end point, when you've collapsed as far as you can go, you're going to straighten back up.

Begin with the lowest vertebra in your back. Vertebra by vertebra, begin to straighten, slowly bringing your back into a vertical position. Move slowly, starting with your lower back. Move up, straightening your mid-back. Then move into your neck, straightening it until your head elongates. Finally, you're in vertical alignment. It will feel as if all of your vertebrae are stacked one on top of another.

Now imagine that there's an invisible thread at the top of your head, pulling you up to the sky, so that your whole vertebral column becomes even more elongated and extends upwards. Also, be aware of sensations in your chest, and see if there's a sense of openness or expansion, maybe even something you identify with pride. The idea is not to fight the collapse, but to allow it to move through to its own completion.

Phase 10 — Uncoupling Fear from the Immobility Response

Preparation

When animals go into immobility because of threat, their response is time-limited.

When they come out of immobility, the locked energy is available for either flight or counter-attack. As humans, we often find that the energy locked in the immobility response is so strong that we're frightened by it. The key to completing this uncompleted immobility response lies in uncoupling our fear from the response itself. This allows the stuck energy to be freed up for use wherever it is needed within the body.

The forces underlying the immobility response and the traumatic emotions of terror, rage, and helplessness are ultimately biological energies. How we access and integrate this energy determines whether we will continue to be frozen and overwhelmed, or we will move through it and thaw. We have a lot going for us; we *can* conquer our fears. With the full use of our highly developed ability to think and perceive, we can, through the felt sense, consciously move out of the trauma response. This process needs to occur gradually rather than abruptly; it is best to take one small phase at a time.

The drive to complete the freezing response remains active no matter how long it has been in place. When we learn how to harness the power of this drive, it becomes our greatest ally in working through the symptoms of trauma. The drive is persistent. Even if we do not do things perfectly, it will always be there to give us another chance. The key is to uncouple fear from the biological immobility response so that the response can complete itself—work through into a meaningful course of action.

Practice
Listen to the exercise on Track Ten of the CD.

LISTEN TO TRACK TEN
Uncoupling Fear from the
Immobility Response

FOURTH GROUP — COMPLETION:
RETURNING TO EQUILIBRIUM

Now that we've discharged stuck energy using the previous group of exercises, we are able to return to equilibrium. But this sense of equilibrium is not something we're used to, so we need to cultivate it.

Orientation plays a critical role in being in the present and in social engagement. When we first come out of our fight or flight responses, we come back to the here and now and make meaningful contact with the objects and organisms in our environment. Often, though, we're so unused to a sense of stillness that we don't know what to make of it.

For someone who's been traumatized, that feeling of balance and wholeness is such a surprise, it can cause an "identity crisis." We don't recognize ourselves because we're no longer filled with shame and fear and collapse.

As you feel equilibrium begin to return, I suggest you use this affirmation: simply say to yourself two or three times, "Home, home at last." Remember that this place of balance and presence is ultimately the place where each of us belongs.

Phase 11 — Orientation: Moving from Internal to External Environment and Social Engagement

Preparation

When we're in trauma, we're not able to be in the present—to see, hear, smell, and perceive our immediate environments fully. As your nervous system begins to return to balance, your orienting responses will naturally begin to come back on line. This next exercise will help that process.

LISTEN TO TRACK ELEVEN

Orientation: Moving from Internal to External Environment and Social Engagement

Practice

During all the previous exercises, you've tended to be focused on what's going on inside of you. As you re-do some of them, or whenever you are doing any kind of body awareness or body sensing exercises, practice the following: As you come back into the outer world and your eyes open, just let your eyes do what they want to do, to look around, to orient. That's the basic nervous system organization that allows for interest, curiosity, and exploration. It's also the antidote for the trauma response.

The nervous system cannot be exploratory, curious, searching, looking, and be traumatized at the same time. Trauma cannot co-exist with these responses. Also, if there is another person around, as you come back from doing one of these internal exercises, you may feel the beginning of an urge to make contact with the person, or simply to look at him or her. That is, again, a natural response. When we're not in the traumatized lock-down mode, our natural response is to reach out and make contact—both with our natural environment and with individuals that we have a relationship with. In the words of a Motown song, "It takes one to stand in the dark alone ... it takes two to let the light shine through."

Phase 12 — Settling and Integrating

Preparation

As you come out of the trauma response, you'll need tools to help draw you into a new sense of presence and calm. The following exercises can be very helpful in helping you settle into your body and into the present moment. I'd like to share with you an affirmation from the Native American tradition: "I give thanks for help unknown, already on its way." Whenever you begin to feel lost or frightened, this affirmation can have a beneficial effect.

Practice

LISTEN TO TRACK TWELVE
Settling and Integrating

This series of postures helps you to calm down after being aroused. Practice the grounding exercise (Phase 2), then follow the sequence pictured, staying in each pose for as long as it is comfortable for you to do so. After each pose, allow time for settling. Notice any changes in your heartbeat and breathing. If you experience shaking or trembling, allow it to happen. I suggest that you look at these pictures and practice the postures whenever you feel agitated or uncomfortable in some way. You can also use the postures as a way of settling so that you can drift into a deeper sleep at night—a sleep that allows you to rest, to restore, and also to give you dreams to further draw you along on your healing journey.

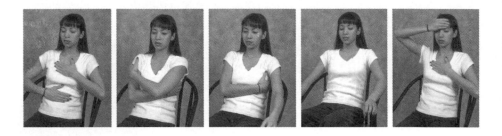

CHAPTER
FIVE

Memory is the selection of images; some elusive, others printed indelibly on the brain. Each image is like a thread ... each thread woven together to make a tapestry of intricate textures. And the tapestry tells a story. And the story is our past ... Like others before me, I have the gift of sight. But the truth changes color depending on the light. And tomorrow can be clearer than yesterday.

—From the film *Eve's Bayou*, screenplay by Kasi Lemmons

Sexual Trauma: Healing the Sacred Wound

IT'S A SHOCKING STATISTIC: Worldwide, one in four persons has been sexually assaulted in childhood. And that's just the conservative estimate! For females, the likelihood is even greater. Of course, we can only speculate how many people are violated as adults. Sexual trauma is clearly one of society's most serious unresolved issues.

In addition, sexual trauma can stem from things other than experiencing direct assault as a child. We may forget, or be unaware of, how prevalent it is to be sexually traumatized by events that generally not thought of as traumatizing.

Consider, for example, gynecological procedures. When performed roughly and insensitively, these can cause the vital organs and energy systems in our pelvis and abdominal organs to go into a kind of shock, not unlike what happens to victims of sexual assault. Even roughly administered thermometers and enemas in childhood can be emotionally injurious.

Abortions can be, and frequently are, traumatizing, as are other invasive surgeries performed to the sexual and internal organs. All or any of these "violations" can cause loss of vitality, diminished capacity for erotic connection and pleasure, and other symptoms of trauma.

We are now seeing significant scientific research showing the detrimental effects of childhood sexual abuse and trauma. As the abused child grows, matures, and then moves through adulthood, a variety of psychological, relational, and/or physical problems inevitably develop.

DEALING WITH SEXUAL TRAUMA

Trauma and sexual abuse are two of our most pressing human and societal problems. They must be studied by unbiased scientific investigation, rather than polarized by hysteria and politics. Millions of people have been tragically hurt by sexual trauma, and we need both scientific study and compassionate application of this knowledge to understand, prevent, and heal trauma.

All sexual trauma is about violation. The consequences of this violation may take the form of:

- Intrusion into our sacred space
- Rupture of personal, emotional, sexual, and energetic boundaries
- A shock to our delicate internal organs
- Feeling soiled, dirty, damaged
- Deep, unexplainable feelings of shame and guilt
- The inability to form deep, sustaining relationships
- A sense of being frozen or shut down

- Overwhelming emotions such as rage, hate, and terror
- Feelings of extreme isolation—a sense of not feeling connected to one's environment, to the human race and to one's self

TRAUMA AND ATTACHMENT

Trauma causes us to have an internal experience that is frightening, angry, and shameful. When we feel threatened, as we do when we are traumatized, our entire organism is geared up to find the *source* of that threat and to do something about it. So it seems natural to look outside of ourselves for the source of that threat. Any animal, when threatened, will locate and identify the source of the threat, will run away from it toward a source of escape and safety.

Young mammals, however, rather than running away from threat, will run towards a source of adult protection, usually to the mother. Similarly, human infants and toddlers will cling to their attachment figures when they feel threatened. However, there is one critically important difference between adult animals and humans: humans *of all ages* seek the comfort of others when we are fearful or stressed.

I think you can see that a dilemma of profound consequences is set up if the people who are supposed to love and protect us are also the ones that hurt, humiliate, and violate us. This sets up a double bind that undermines people's basic sense of self and trust in their own instincts. Our sense of safety and stability in the world and our interpersonal relationships becomes undermined by childhood abuse because we carry these early thwarted—that is deeply conflicted—survival patterns into adulthood.

TRANSFORMING THE LEGACY

It doesn't help matters that we live in such a sex-negative culture. What generally gets overlooked is that sexual energy and life-force energy are virtually one and the same. People who have passion for life have a flow of creative energy that feels inspiring and uplifting to be around. It is life-positive. They are considered to be "juicy." Those around them soak up their spark and creative exuberance. Instead of being the norm, they stand out. Why is that? And what is creative life force anyway? Where does it originate?

In Indian culture, it is referred to as "second chakra energy," and it arises from our sexual organs. It is the arousal energy that made troubadours sing, the great masters compose, build, paint, create theater, and write literature that delights us and endures through time. It is the energy of both creation and procreation.

Unfortunately, so much fear exists about this potent force that social and religious institutions have had a pervasive influence in damping it down. When a lid is put on feelings and sensations that are normal, they become pathologized. Instead of acceptance, it is difficult for living, breathing human beings to know what to do with these feelings. Any attempt to dictate what thoughts, feelings, and sensations are proper or improper creates a breeding ground for guilt and shame.

Thoughts are thoughts and sensations are sensations. Period! They do not need to be acted out inappropriately. When the moral judgment is removed, individuals are able to acknowledge and experience their authentic life energy freely. Healthy decisions and expressions of sexuality are more likely when the defensive mechanisms of denial and repression are no longer necessary. The unspeakable becomes spoken, and families can become a model for shaping healthy, instead of damaging, behavior.

HEALTHY SEXUALITY

Let's look at two critical stages of child development: early childhood and adolescence. Somewhere between the ages of four and six, children feel a special bond and attraction to their opposite sex parent. In fact, this phenomenon is so universal that the Greeks portrayed the unfortunate consequences of this *unresolved* dilemma in the plays *Oedipus Rex* and *Electra*. (Of course, with new, blended and same-sex households, these stages may show up differently.)

Daughters, especially around the age of five, routinely "fall in love" with their dads, as do little boys with their moms. This is a normal, healthy stage of development. Children of this age will "flirt" with the parent of the opposite sex. This is not flirting in the adult, sexual sense, but rather a developmental "practicing." In other words, the kinds of behaviors that will later form the repertoire of adolescent, peer flirtations are first elicited and tested at home where it is supposed to be safe. This is the time when little girls will tell their fathers, "I love you, Daddy. I want to marry you and have a baby."

At this delicate, vulnerable age, what is needed to foster healthy development is for the father to tenderly say (and mean) something like: "I love you too, sweetheart, but Daddy's married to Mommy. When you grow up you can marry someone special just for you and, if you want, you can have children with him."

Often, what happens instead, is that the child's behavior may be handled poorly by misreading this innocent (and it *is* truly innocent) practicing. Instead of the response being that of a parent helping the child with his or her emerging sexuality, the response may resemble something more like that of a lover, promoting their "special" relationship. Playful flirtations can then result in awkward and inappropriate responses by the parent. This "courting" behavior can be quite confusing and often feels overwhelming to the child and may be frightening to the parent as well. This is a place where well-defined generational boundaries are so important and frequently are weak in adults who were themselves sexually traumatized as children.

If these lessons are not learned early on, it is likely that a sudden fracture of the parent-child relationship will occur at the next important stage of sexual development—adolescence. At this time the parent is confronted with a blossoming young lady or man who looks like the spouse that he/she fell in love with some years earlier—but perhaps even more beautiful or handsome. If the parents are not comfortable with their own sexuality and warmly erotic with each other, this sudden attraction to their teenager may cause what's known as *incest panic.*

Particularly in the case of father-daughter relationships, the father is drawn to his offspring in ways that the possibility of acting them out seems real and threatening. Out of this fear, he suddenly cuts off physical warmth and becomes distant and cold. In this typical scenario, the daughter feels not only abandoned but also rejected because of her new and fragile sexuality and forming sense of self.

And then there is the possibility that at different ages, the father may have actually acted out sexually with her. He may have touched her inappropriately or kissed her on the mouth, with a more adult kiss. This could have frightened daughter and father both. And, tragically, in some cases it goes farther.

So how can these awkward, but common (if not inevitable) sexual feelings be handled? If we repress these "unthinkable" feelings, they can build like pressure in a volcano, later to be felt covertly by the youngster as tension within the family relationships. What are the options? Held in, these powerful energies can create perversions, including frigidity, impotence, and symptoms such as addictions and health problems. Acted out in sexual ways, they can become promiscuity.

REGULATING YOUR SEXUAL FEELINGS

None of the above choices is appealing to healthy individuals. Let's take a look at a refreshing approach. With honesty, compassion, and using the felt sense you learned working with the Twelve-Phase Healing Trauma Program, you can regulate these energies. First of all when these sensations arise, notice them for what they are and try to accept them in a non-shaming way as part of a shared, if not universal, human experience.

Next, allow these sensations to pendulate and move through as waves of pure energy. The energy is then free to be expressed in creative outlets or transferred to an appropriate partner. These conflicts can be moved through in a surprisingly short time.

Here is a simple case example to illustrate this point. I helped a young father who was terrified to diaper his infant son. As we worked together, I had him focus on the sensations that arose without thought or judgment. As he did this, the sexual sensations turned to anger as he remembered that as a very young boy he had been molested by his favorite grandfather. These sensations allowed him to feel anger toward his grandfather for the first time. As the anger slowly dissolved, tears of liberation flowed. He was relieved to know that he wasn't a bad person.

At home, he noticed his sensations as he watched his wife change his son. He was pleased at how quickly the sexual sensations that he felt became directed toward his wife instead, and as he gazed at his little boy the feelings that emerged were those of love, care, and pride.

In summary, when parents become less afraid of experiencing their own sensations, practice appropriate boundaries, and have an understanding of what children need to develop healthy sexuality, awkwardness and tension turn into more comfortable familial relationships. Parents then become free to show warmth and affection to their children—at any developmental stage—in ways that are neither romanticized nor sexualized.

When puberty hits, teenagers are less likely either to feel inept with their own love relationships, only to be compulsively driven into promiscuity in an attempt to get their needs for love met that a rejecting repressed parent wasn't able to give, *or* to re-enact a violation of their sexual boundaries. In this way, the cycle of intergenerational sexual trauma can be interrupted, and a new legacy of life-positive energy can be passed on.

Finally, I wish to acknowledge the reality that many successful families have two parents of the same sex, and that even more are single-parent families. Though your family may not fit the heterosexual, two-parent model I've presented here, I trust that some of the ideas I've presented will have relevance to your situation as well.

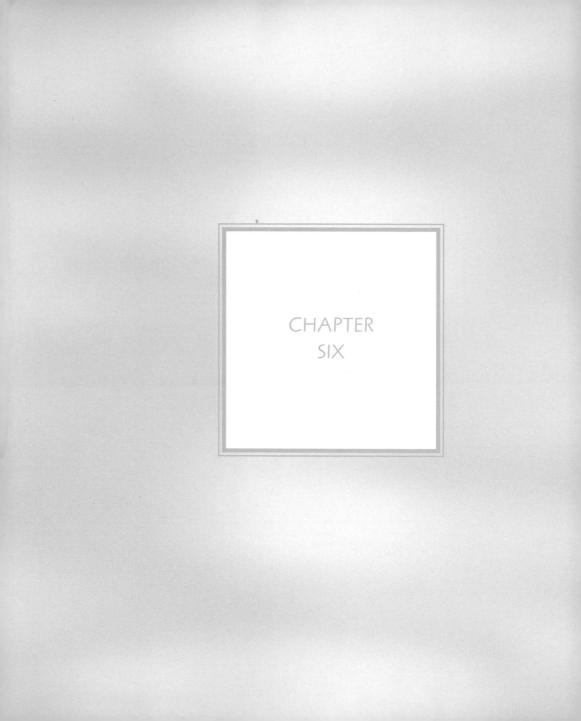

CHAPTER
SIX

You lose yourself, you reappear,
You suddenly find you got nothing to fear.
—Bob Dylan

Spirituality and Trauma: Pathway to Awakening

ACCORDING TO SEVERAL Buddhist and Taoist traditions, sex, meditation, death, and trauma share a common potential. These are *the great portals*—catalysts for profound surrender and awakening. Unfortunately, most of us are not prepared to take the opportunities offered by these powerful teachers.

Let's take a look at sex first. Though many of us have experienced glimpses of sexual ecstasy, the focus on titillation, seduction, and performance in post-Viagra America often obscure the possibility for deep emotional and spiritual surrender that sex can offer.

Meditation is another avenue to awakening, but because of the years of dedication required to achieve what many of the great traditions refer to as "ego-death" through meditative practice, very few people have succeeded using this method.

The process of dying, a final chance to make peace with ourselves, has been given over largely to doctors, drugs, and machines. Even in supportive and conscious settings, what should be a spiritual act of surrender at the time of death is too often overshadowed by the sad remorse that the surrender did not occur earlier in life.

SURRENDER AND TRANSFORMATION

Trauma is the fourth pathway to awakening. In transforming and releasing ourselves from trauma we must face, as does the newborn child, an uncertain world. It is a world stripped of the illusion of safety, and it obliges us to learn an entirely new way of being. When we enter it, we soon discover that our instinctive energies are not limited to acts of flight or uncontrolled violence. They are our *heroic energies*. And they can be harnessed! The energies that are released when we heal from trauma are the wellspring of our creative, artistic, and poetic sensibilities, and they can be summoned to propel us into the wholeness of our intelligence.

Trauma is about thwarted instincts. Instincts, by definition, are always in the present. When we allow them their rightful domain, we surrender to the "eternal now." With the full presence of mind and body, we can gain access to the source of our own energy and enthusiasm. Consider for a moment the word *enthusiasm*. It comes from the Greek words *en*, meaning within, and *Theos*, meaning God. When we reclaim our enthusiasm for life, we are drawing closer to God, becoming more spiritual.

As we resolve our traumas, we discover missing parts of our beings, those that make us feel whole and complete. Our instincts house the simple but vital knowledge that "I am I," and "I am here." Without this sense of belonging in the world, we are lost, disconnected from life. If we learn how to surrender to our inborn knowledge, it can lead us on a healing journey that will bring us face to face with our natural spirituality, our God-given connection to life.

The process of healing trauma can drop us into virtual birth canals of consciousness. From these vantage points, we can position ourselves to be propelled fully into the stream of life. Healing from trauma can be that final instinctive push, that inner shaking and trembling, "the kick," that can awaken us and lead us on a journey home.

This mythical inner adventure can be likened to being on a raft in unfamiliar waters. The first thing we notice is that we can't simply think our way down the river. Our rational minds are not equipped to operate the craft by themselves. We need paddles. We need our bodies, our instincts, to maneuver and steer it. We begin to feel the power in our arms as we engage our instinctive "felt sense."

As we gain confidence in our ability to handle the raft, we are ready to ride the rapids that lead us into a deathlike cavern, the frozen world in which we feel helpless and unable to move. Suddenly, we no longer can move, or even breathe. All of our senses heighten simultaneously, but this time we are *not* helpless. We are no longer bound to relive the overwhelming nightmare of the original event. We are neither stuck in the past, nor are we consumed by feelings of pending doom, or by fanciful daydreams of the future. We are here, now. Our instinctive awareness keeps us in the present, in the flow. Our paddles, our body energy, propel us through the deathlike icy darkness until we re-emerge into the sunlight. In the warmth, we reconnect with life.

We are awakened to a new self, and to a New World. With gentle and appropriate guidance, we can successfully navigate the troubled waters of our traumas. We can learn, as well, how to guide each other through the nightmares created by these altered states, and reconnect with the stream of life.

In this book, we've looked at the suffering that unresolved trauma can cause, and the hope for healing that exists for each one of us. Using the techniques of the Twelve-Phase Healing Trauma Program, anyone can begin to break through the bonds of unresolved trauma and live in a fuller, more deeply fulfilling way. The trauma that once stopped us in our tracks can become instead the very key that unlocks a great transformation. I wish you the very best in your healing journey, wherever it may take you.

Helpful Tips and Techniques for Preventing Trauma

TRAUMATIC EXPERIENCES are an unavoidable fact of life. At some point, it's almost inevitable that a family member or friend will suffer an accident or other traumatic experience. However, there are many ways to help that person to prevent long-term trauma from developing. This section provides hints and tips for working with someone who has had a traumatic experience, with specific guidance on how to work with children as well as adults. Always use your own best judgment to assess the particular circumstances with which you are dealing. What are given here are simply guidelines to help loved ones.

FIRST AID FOR ADULTS

STAGE I: IMMEDIATE ACTION (AT THE SCENE OF THE ACCIDENT)
If life-saving medical procedures are required, of course that must take precedence.

Encourage a sense of safety. Keep the person warm, lying down, and still, unless, of course, they face further danger remaining where they are. Don't let them jump up, which they may be tempted to do. The feeling of having to do something, to act in some way, can override the essential need for stillness and the discharge of energy. They may want to deny the magnitude of the accident, and might act like they are fine.

Stay with the injured person. Assure them that you will stay with them, or that help is on the way. When help does arrive, continue to stay with the injured person, if possible.

Encourage the person to fully experience their bodily sensations. These may include adrenaline rush, numbness, shaking and trembling, feeling hot or chilled. (Of course, you can only do this if the accident is not too serious.)

Stay fully present. What you do and say can help the person discharge. Let them know it is not only okay that they shake, but it is good and will help them release the shock. They will get a sense of relief after the shaking is completed and may feel warmth in their hands and feet. Their breathing should be fuller and easier. This initial stage could easily take fifteen to twenty minutes.

Don't go it alone. If necessary, get someone to help *you* process the event afterwards.

STAGE II: ONCE THE PERSON IS MOVED HOME OR TO THE HOSPITAL

Allow time for processing. Continue to keep the injured person quiet and resting until they are out of the acute shock reaction. Injured people should always take a day or two off work to allow themselves to reintegrate. This is important even if they perceive that the injury doesn't justify staying home. This resistance can be a common denial mechanism and defense from feelings of helplessness.

Common injuries, such as whiplash, will compound and require *much* longer healing times if this initial recovery stage is bypassed. A day or two of rest is good insurance.

Allow the emotions to be felt without judgment. The accident survivor is likely to begin experiencing a variety of emotions, such as anger, fear, grief, guilt, anxiety. There might also be bodily sensations, such as shaking, chills, etc. This is still fine.

STAGE III: BEGINNING TO ACCESS AND RENEGOTIATE THE TRAUMA

This stage often coincides with Stage II, and is essential for accessing the stored energy of trauma so that it can be fully released. It is important to help people recall the peripheral images, feelings, and sensations they experienced, not just those directly related to the event.

Focus on sensations. Throughout any of these stages, be aware that as people talk about their experiences, they may become activated or agitated. Their breathing may change and become more rapid. Their heart rate might increase, or they might break into a sweat. If this happens, stop talking about the experience and focus on what sensations they are having in their body, such as, "I have a pain in my neck," or "I feel sick to my stomach." If you are not sure, ask them what they are feeling.

Let the energy discharge. When the people appear calmed and relaxed, move into a more detailed account of the experience and the sensations. They may notice some slight shaking and trembling. Assure them that this is natural. Point out that the activation response is decreasing and that you are working slowly to bring the energy up and discharge it. This process is known as *titration*—taking one small step at a time.

TRAUMA PREVENTION FOR CHILDREN

Of all the trauma-producing events that can cause physical symptoms and emotional problems later in life, medical procedures are potentially the most damaging. Many clinics unintentionally amplify the fear of an already frightened child. In preparation for some routine procedures, infants are strapped into "papooses" to keep them from moving. A child that struggles so much that he or she needs to be tied down, however, is a child too frightened to be restrained without suffering the consequences. Likewise, a child who is severely frightened is not a good candidate for anesthesia until a sense of tranquility has been restored. A child induced into anesthesia while frightened will almost certainly be traumatized, often severely. Children can even be traumatized by insensitively administered enemas or thermometers.

Much of the trauma associated with medical procedures can be prevented if health care providers do the following:

- Encourage parents to stay with their children
- Explain as much as possible in advance
- Delay procedures until the children are calm

The problem is that few professionals understand trauma or the lasting and pervasive effects these procedures can have. Although medical personnel are often quite concerned with the children's welfare, they may need more information from you, the consumer.

HOW TO HELP A TRAUMATIZED CHILD

When your child has experienced a traumatic event, remembering these steps will support him or her in resolving the trauma:

Focus on your own reactions. Assuming that there is no imminent danger, take a moment to observe your own internal physiological and emotional responses until *you* settle and have a sense of relative calm.

Pay attention to your child's bodily responses and words. Validate your child's bodily responses by not interrupting the trembling, shaking, or tears that are a normal part of coming out of shock.

Support these reactions. You can do this by demonstrating your acceptance through words and/or touch. For example, put one hand on your child's shoulder, arm, or middle of the back. Use a reassuring voice to say a few words, such as, "That's okay," "It's all right to cry" (feel angry, and so on), or "Just let the shaking happen."

Be there for the child. After the trembling, shaking, or tears stop, validate your child's emotional responses. Let him or her know that whatever they are feeling is okay and you will stay and listen to him or her. Resist the temptation to talk them out of fear, sadness, anger, embarrassment, guilt or shame in order to avoid your own uncomfortable feelings. Trust that your child will move these feelings, supported by your acceptance of his or her authentic self.

Revisit the experience later. When helping your child move through symptoms developed from an earlier experience, you can use drawings, stories, and play to elicit movement of residual trauma energy that may be stuck. Generally the adult needs to tell the story of what he or she believes happened, then invite the child to add their version. Sometimes it is best to use a different name for the child in the story. This may help initially to give needed distance from the event. You may also want to reintroduce your child to ordinary objects or experiences that remain "charged" because they in some way remind the child of the incident that overwhelmed them.

After an automobile accident, for example, the infant's or toddler's car seat could be brought into the living room. Holding the infant in your arms, or gently walking with the toddler, you can gradually move toward it together and eventually place the child in the seat.

Go slowly. The key here is to take baby steps, watching and waiting for responses such as stiffening, turning away, holding the breath, or heart rate changes. With each gentle approach to the avoided or fear-provoking encounter, the same procedure outlined above can be used as a guide. The idea is to make sure that your pacing is in tune with your child's needs so that not too much energy or emotion is released at once. You can tell if this is occurring if the child seems to be getting more wound up. Calm your child by offering gentle reassurance, touching, holding, or rocking.

Use play for healing. Puppets, dolls, or miniature toy figures can also be useful in assessing if any trauma indications exist, and can help your child move through them. For example, when a child's physical body has recovered after surgery, a miniature bed and play figures that include a child, mom, dad, doctor, and nurse can be given to the child to play with. Watch your child's reactions closely. With the suggestions you've learned in this chapter, gently guide your child to sense his or her body's reactions and release any uncomfortable feelings.

HOW CAN I TELL IF MY CHILD HAS BEEN TRAUMATIZED?

Any unusual behavior that begins shortly after a severely frightening episode or medical procedure, particularly with anesthesia, may indicate that your child is traumatized. Compulsive, repetitive mannerisms—such as repeatedly smashing a toy car into a doll—are an almost sure sign of an unresolved reaction to a traumatic event. The activity may or may not be a literal replay of the trauma. Other signs of traumatic stress include:

- Persistent, controlling behaviors
- Regression to earlier behavior patterns, such as thumb-sucking
- Tantrums, uncontrollable rage attacks
- Hyperactivity
- Tendency to startle easily
- Recurring night terrors or nightmares
- Thrashing while asleep
- Bed-wetting
- Inability to concentrate in school, forgetfulness
- Excessive belligerence or shyness, withdrawal or fearfulness
- Extreme need to cling
- Stomachaches, headaches, or other ailments of unknown origin

To find out whether an uncustomary behavior is indeed a traumatic reaction, try mentioning the frightening episode and see how your child responds. A traumatized child may not want to be reminded of the predisposing event, or conversely, once reminded, will become excited or fearful and unable to stop talking about it.

It's also important to realize that children who have outgrown unusual behavior patterns have not necessarily discharged the energy that gave rise to them. The reason traumatic reactions can hide for years is that the maturing nervous system is able to control the excess energy. By reminding your child of a frightening incident that precipitated altered behaviors in years past, you may well stir up signs of traumatic residue.

Reactivating a traumatic symptom need not be cause for concern. The physiological processes involved, primitive as they are, respond well to interventions that both engage and allow them to follow the natural course of healing. Children are wonderfully receptive to experiencing the healing side of a traumatic reaction. Your job is simply to provide an opportunity for this to occur. A few minutes spent with your child in an appropriate way can not only minimize the chance of lasting effects, but actually make the child more resilient to life's stresses and later extreme events.

Additional Resources

FOR MORE INFORMATION on this approach, known as Somatic Experiencing® and Peter A. Levine's work through the Foundation for Human Enrichment, please visit www.traumahealing.com online, or email info@traumahealing.com. On the traumahealing.com web site, you can access information about Peter A. Levine's teaching schedule, as well as a directory of practitioners trained by the Foundation for Human Enrichment.

For further reading on the subject of healing trauma, see Peter A. Levine's *Waking the Tiger: Healing Trauma: The Innate Capacity to Transform Overwhelming Experiences* (North Atlantic Books, 1997).

If you believe that your healing journey would benefit from consultation with a trained therapist, there are many local resources that can help you find an appropriate professional to work with. Remember, you are the consumer: don't be afraid to ask potential therapists questions about their training, background, and experience in working with trauma.

About the Author

PETER A. LEVINE received his Ph.D. in medical biophysics from the University of California at Berkeley, and also holds a doctorate in psychology from International University. He has worked in the field of stress and trauma for 35 years, and is the developer of Somatic Experiencing.® He provides training in this work throughout the world. He has taught and spent time in various indigenous cultures internationally, including time at the Hopi Guidance Center in Second Mesa, Arizona. Peter has been stress consultant for NASA in the development of the first space shuttle. He is a member of the Institute of World Affairs Task Force with Psychologists for Social Responsibility and serves on the American Psychological Association initiative for response to large-scale disaster and ethno-political warfare. He is on the distinguished faculty of Santa Barbara Graduate Institute. Peter is the author of the bestselling book, *Waking the Tiger: Healing Trauma,* which has been published in thirteen languages, as well as three audio learning series for Sounds True.

CD SESSIONS

FIRST GROUP—PREPARATORY PHASES

1. Safety and Containment Exercises: Finding Your Body Boundaries

2. Grounding and Centering

3. Building Resources

SECOND GROUP—TRACKING SKILLS

4. From "Felt Sense" to Tracking Specific Sensations

5. Tracking Activation: Sensations, Images, Thoughts, and Emotions

6. Pendulation: Tracking Your Rhythms of Expansion and Contraction

THIRD GROUP—DISCHARGING ACTIVATION

7. Fight Response: Natural Aggression versus Violence

8. Flight Response: Natural Escape versus Anxiety

9. Strength and Resiliency versus Collapse and Defeat

10. Uncoupling Fear from the Immobility Response

FOURTH GROUP—COMPLETION: RETURNING TO EQUILIBRIUM

11. Orientation: Moving from Internal to External Environment
and Social Engagement

12. Settling and Integrating